Tonsils and Adenoids

Edited by Balwant Singh Gendeh

Published in London, United Kingdom

Tonsils and Adenoids
http://dx.doi.org/10.5772/intechopen.12341
Edited by Balwant Singh Gendeh

Contributors
Georgios Giourgos, Alberto Luchena, Chiara Bovi, Hardip Singh Gendeh, Balwant Singh Gendeh, Anubhuti Dhanuka, Anukaran Mahajan, Karunesh Gupta, Stuti Mahajan, Sebastiano Bucolo, Matteo Pezzoli, Maria Vittoria Pomara, Umberto Visentin, Gianni Succo, Du-Bois Asante, Patrick Kafui Akakpo, Gideon Akuamoah Wiafe, Anusha Vaddi, Shravan Renapurkar, Sonam Khurana

First published in London, United Kingdom, 2023 by IntechOpen
IntechOpen is the global imprint of INTECHOPEN LIMITED, registered in England and Wales, registration number: 11086078, 5 Princes Gate Court, London, SW7 2QJ, United Kingdom

British Library Cataloguing-in-Publication Data
A catalogue record for this book is available from the British Library

Additional hard and PDF copies can be obtained from orders@intechopen.com

Tonsils and Adenoids
Edited by Balwant Singh Gendeh
p. cm.
Print ISBN 978-1-83769-535-5
Online ISBN 978-1-83769-534-8
eBook (PDF) ISBN 978-1-83769-536-2

Meet the editor

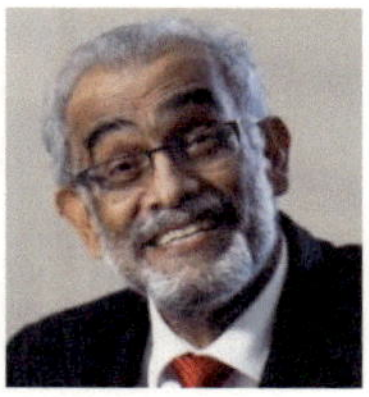

Dr. Balwant Singh Gendeh is a senior consultant ENT surgeon with a subspeciality interest in rhinology. His previous achievements include being an ENT registrar at the Royal Infirmary, Middlesbrough, UK in 1993 and a Fulbright Scholar to the United States in 1997 at the University of Pittsburgh Medical Centre (UPMC), Hospital University of Pennsylvania (HUP), Philadelphia, and St. Joseph's Hospital, Chicago. He received a diploma from the Fellowship Academy of Medicine Malaysia (FAMM) in 2000. He was the previous board chairman of the Malaysian American Commission on Educational Exchange (MACEE), an international fellow of the American Academy of Otolaryngology-Head and Neck Surgery (AAOHNS), and a fellow of the Academy of Sciences Malaysia (FASc). Dr. Gendeh has written and published ninety-eight scientific papers and thirty-eight book chapters and edited ten books.

Contents

Preface

This book discusses selected topics on the tonsils and adenoids, providing insight into advancements in the field. The book includes the following six chapters:

Chapter 1: "Therapeutic Approaches in Chronic Adenoiditis"

Chapter 2: "Peritonsillar and Intratonsillar Abscess: A Review on Clinical Features, Managements and Complications"

Chapter 3: "Evolution of Adenoid Surgery"

Chapter 4: "3D Exoscopic Surgery (3Des) for Tonsillectomy"

Chapter 5: "The Link between Adenoids and Nasopharyngeal Carcinoma"

Chapter 6: "Benign and Malignant Tumors of the Tonsils"

The chapters present new clinical and research developments as well as future perspectives on the many types of problems and lesions of the tonsils and adenoids. It is a useful resource for ENT surgeons, laryngologists, head and neck surgeons, rhinologists, chest physicians, general physicians, postgraduates, research trainees, and general practitioners with a special interest in pharynx and related problems.

I would like to thank and congratulate the chapter authors for their excellent contributions and the time taken in writing the chapters. I would also like to thank the valuable teachers from whom I have gained knowledge throughout the years. I am grateful to IntechOpen for giving me the opportunity to serve as editor for this book. My sincere thanks go to Author Service Manager Zrinka Tomicic for guiding me through the publication process and moving the book ahead in a timely fashion and to the technical editors for arranging the book in a uniform format.

I dedicate this book to my spouse, children, and loved ones for all their patience and understanding.

Balwant Singh Gendeh, MBBS, MS(ORL-HNS),UKM, AM(Mal), FAMM, FASc (M'sia), FMSA
Retired Professor,
Department of Otorhinolaryngology, Head and Neck Surgery,
Universiti Kebangsaan Medical Center,
Cheras, Malaysia

Senior Consultant,
ENT Resident Surgeon (Rhinology – Allergy, Endoscopic Sinus and Skull Base Surgery, Functional and Cosmetic Nasal Surgery),
Pantai Hospital,
Kuala Lumpur, Malaysia

Chapter 1

Therapeutic Approaches in Chronic Adenoiditis

Georgios Giourgos, Alberto Luchena and Chiara Bovi

Abstract

Adenoid tissue diseases (acute adenoiditis, adenoid hypertrophy, and chronic adenoiditis) typically occur in childhood. Adenoid hypertrophy seems to be related to many factors, such as infections, passive smoking, and low vitamin D levels, while the role of allergy still remains controversial. Chronic adenoiditis incidence has increased in recent years, as a result of higher rates of upper airway infections and biofilm formation, with multiple potential clinical complications. Diagnosis is typically clinical, with physical examination and nasal endoscopy. The treatment can be medical or surgical. Non-surgical treatment of chronic adenoiditis with intranasal steroids and leukotriene inhibitors has proven to be effective, reducing the size of the adenoid tissue and symptoms. On the other hand, adenoidectomy is one of the commonest ENT surgical procedures with excellent outcomes and rare adverse events. Curettage adenoidectomy is widely used by many ENT surgeon, but presents risk of residual adenoidal tissue, especially in peritubaric and superior nasopharynx regions. In the last years, different surgical techniques have been proposed to reduce surgical risk and morbidity, such as electrocautery adenoidectomy, microdebrider adenoidectomy, and coblation adenoidectomy. Intranasal or transoral endoscopes enabled a great control of surgical field and a complete removal of adenoid tissue.

Keywords: adenoids, adenoid hypertrophy, adenoidectomy, coblation, suction diathermy, microdebrider

1. Introduction

The adenoids or nasopharyngeal tonsils are aggregates of lymphoid tissue located at the posterior wall of the nasopharynx, at the level of the soft palate. Together with the lingual and palatine tonsils they form the Waldeyer's ring, providing an immediate barrier against upper respiratory tract infections and promoting immunity against microorganisms from outside [1].

Histologically, they are composed of epithelial cells, lymphocytes, macrophages, and dendritic cells [2]. Adenoids as well as tonsils are composed mainly of B lymphocytes (50–65%), while T cell lymphocytes comprise 40% of all adenoid and tonsillar lymphocytes. Only 3% is represented by mature plasma cells [3].

The adenoids are present at birth, develop progressively throughout childhood, and reach their maximum size at about age seven. They then decrease in size due to physiological atrophy during puberty, becoming almost absent by adulthood.

Adenoiditis is therefore a typical disease in childhood and adolescence [1].

2. Adenoiditis

Adenoiditis occurs when there is inflammation of the adenoid tissue resulting from infection, allergies, or inflammation such as irritation from stomach acid as a component of laryngopharyngeal reflux (LPR) [1].

It can be distinguished in acute adenoiditis, adenoid hypertrophy, and chronic adenoiditis.

2.1 Acute adenoiditis

Acute adenoiditis is often the consequence of a viral upper airway infection, often followed by bacterial overinfection [1]. It presents most frequently with the following symptoms: high fever, severe nasal obstruction, mouth breathing, and yellow snot dripping from the posterior pharyngeal wall. In particular, nasal obstruction in infants can lead to dystithia, increased neutrophils, high C-reactive protein (CRP) levels in the peripheral blood, and enlarged adenoids on the lateral image of the pharynx [4, 5].

2.2 Adenoid hypertrophy/vegetation

Adenoid hypertrophy/vegetation represents the most frequently observed clinical condition in ENT medical practice. Its clinical manifestations include mouth breathing, snoring, and adenoid-face. Typically nasal obstruction gets worse in the supine position, leading to sleep apnea in severe cases (obstructive sleep apnea-hypopnea syndrome or OSAHS) [6]. Factors contributing to sleep apnea include obesity, allergies, asthma, gastroenterological reflux disorder (GERD), abnormalities in the physical structure of the face or jaw, and various medical and neurological conditions [2].

Infections are the main cause of adenoid hypertrophy. Interestingly, Epstein–Barr virus (EBV) and Human Bocavirus (HBoV) have been detected throughout the year in samples of children with asymptomatic chronic adenotonsillar diseases, thus attesting their constant presence in the lymphoepithelial tissues of the upper respiratory tract and a pathogenetic potential for development of lymphoid hypertrophy and chronic inflammation [7].

Passive smoking is one of the most notorious risk factors for airway infections in children, such as pharyngitis, rhinitis, sinusitis, otitis, laryngitis, bronchitis, and pneumonia. It has been evidenced in many studies that cigarette smoking reduces the Th1/Th2 ratio and increases proinflammatory molecules, leading to structural changes in the respiratory nasal mucosa, such as impaired ciliary activity and mucociliary function [8]. Moreover, IFN-γ production by CD8+ T cells is severely reduced, thus promoting respiratory tract infections [9].

A recent study by Shin et al. [10] evidenced the correlation between low vitamin D levels and adenotonsillar hypertrophy, emphasizing the importance in measuring serum 25(OH)D level in children with sleep-disordered breathing (SDB) symptoms and increased sizes of the adenoids and tonsils.

The role of allergy in adenoidal disease is still controversial. Sadeghi-Shabestari et al. [11] demonstrated a significant correlation between a positive skin prick test and the high level of serum IgE in patients with adenotonsillar hypertrophy (ATH) rather than other children, while a study by Modrzynski and Zawisz [12] reported that children with allergic rhinitis appeared to be more susceptible to adenoidal hypertrophy (AH). They showed that adenoid hypertrophy was more frequently represented in children with allergic rhinitis related to hypersensitivity to dust mites, than in children with other allergic diseases (asthma/atopic dermatitis) or with no allergies. Furthermore, a hypersensitivity to plant pollen allergens and mold allergens was more frequent in children with AH than in children without AH, demonstrating the role of allergic rhinitis (AR) as the main cause of allergic inflammation around the adenoid.

Another focus of studies is the relevance of localized allergic response in the nasal mucosa of local allergic rhinitis (LAR), in the absence of systemic atopy [13]. In this regard, it has been evidenced that specific immunoglobulin E (sIgE) antibodies are produced locally [13–15] and the local production of total IgE and sIgE antibodies to Dermatophagoides pteronyssinus (DP) has been demonstrated in the adenoid tissues of atopic children [16].

A recent study by Cho et al. [17] reported a higher sIgE-positive rate in local tissue than in serum. Moreover, 36.2% of children with sIgE-negative serum resulted positive for sIgE in adenotonsillar tissue, suggesting that local allergic inflammation may play an important role in adenotonsillar tissues. These results are in line with a study by Zhang et al. [18] that reported inconsistency in the expression of sIgE antibodies between adenotonsillar tissues and serum.

Furthermore, this study showed that the serum and/or adenotonsillar tissue of 70.6% of children with adenotonsillar hypertrophy (ATH) were sensitized to more than one allergen, suggesting that children with ATH are more likely to have concomitant allergies compared to the general population [17].

However, other studies have found no direct correlation between allergies and adenotonsillar hypertrophy [19–22].

2.3 Chronic adenoiditis

Chronic adenoiditis (**Figure 1**) occurs frequently in children (mainly those aged 3–7 years) [23], showing many of the same manifestations of adenoid hypertrophy, such as continuous or intermittent snoring, mouth breathing, and dry mouth.

However, clinical manifestations, such as fever, increased leucocytes, granulocytes, and elevated CRP levels, are rarely observed when chronic adenoiditis is not severe [6].

Polymicrobial infections and biofilm formation are often the main causes of this chronic disease [24].

A bacterial biofilm (BF) is a membrane-like substance formed by the polysaccharide matrix, fibrous proteins, and proteolipid proteins secreted by bacteria attached to the surfaces of tissues. BFs contain various types of bacteria and even DNA and RNA [25].

The main bacteria are responsible for nasopharyngeal biofilm formation are the otopathogens (*H. influenzae*, *M. catarrhalis*, and *S. pneumoniae*), also leading to middle ear infections [26–30].

It has been suggested that the presence of bacterial biofilm may act as the primary source of infection for other closely related structures, leading to rhinosinusitis, pharyngitis, tonsillitis, and otitis media [24, 31, 32], and may be partially responsible

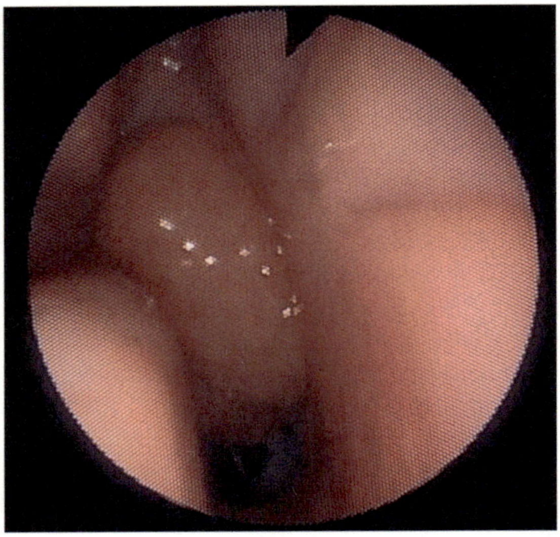

Figure 1.
Chronic adenoiditis.

for the ineffectiveness of traditional antibiotic treatment. This seems to be due to the physical barrier formed by the extracellular matrix, which blocks antibiotic diffusion within the biofilm, as well as some characteristics of the biofilm, such as reduced bacterial replication in the inner layers and resistance mechanisms acquired as a result of the quorum-sensing process [29].

2.3.1 Clinical complications of chronic adenoiditis

Chronic adenoiditis is a long-term infection (especially bacterial infection) that may involve close anatomical structures, leading to acute or chronic infections, such as rhinitis, rhinosinusitis, chronic pharyngitis, cobblestone throat, soft palatitis, abscesses of the posterior pharyngeal wall, and abscesses of the peripharyngeal wall. As observed in all infections, chronic adenoiditis can result in lymphadenitis, typically presenting as an enlargement of the laterocervical and intraglandular-parotid lymph nodes.

Recent studies evidenced that adenoid diseases are one of the main causes of post-nasal drip syndrome (also known as upper airway cough syndrome, UACS) in children, and thus, responsible for chronic cough. Adenoid involvement should be suspected when chronic cough appears or worsens upon postural change or occurs after falling asleep or waking up in the morning.

Moreover, chronic adenoiditis may induce several "infectious immune" diseases, such as rheumatic fever, glomerulonephritis, nephrotic syndrome, and anaphylactoid purpura. Regarding autoimmune nephropathy, it seems that the immune mechanism that causes glomerulonephritis from palatine tonsillitis may be the same as adenoiditis [6].

Given the close relationship between the pharynx and the adenoids with the atlantoaxial joint and the shared venous and lymphatic circulation, an inflammatory involvement of the cervical spine from an upper airway infection has been described. This rare syndrome is known as Grisel's syndrome, presenting with spontaneous luxation or subluxation of the atlas on the axis, secondary to hyperemia and laxity of the atlanto-axial joints [33].

Chronic adenoiditis represents one of the main causes of ozostomia, together with chronic tonsillitis, tonsillar calculus, and gastrointestinal function disorders, such as gastroesophageal reflux and laryngopharyngeal reflux [6].

Chronic or recurrent middle ear disease is a frequent complication of chronic adenoiditis, due to bacterial colonization of the middle ear along the Eustachian tube, inducing suppurative otitis media [34]. Furthermore, adenoid hypertrophy can obstruct the auditory tube, leading to increased tympanic pressure and secretory otitis media [35].

3. Adenoids and middle ear

The adenoids are located on the posterior wall of the nasopharynx, and they may extend laterally to the ostium of the Eustachian tube, creating a close anatomical and functional relationship with the middle ear, and suggesting how chronic adenoiditis may be complicated by the development of chronic or recurrent middle ear disease. Clinical manifestations of middle ear disease include the presence of serous or mucous fluid in the middle ear, persisting for at least 3 months (chronic otitis media with effusion, OME [36]) (**Figures 2** and **3**); repeated acute middle ear infections, with at least three episodes within a period of 6 months or more than four episodes in a period of 12 months (recurrent acute otitis media, RAOM) [37]; long-lasting

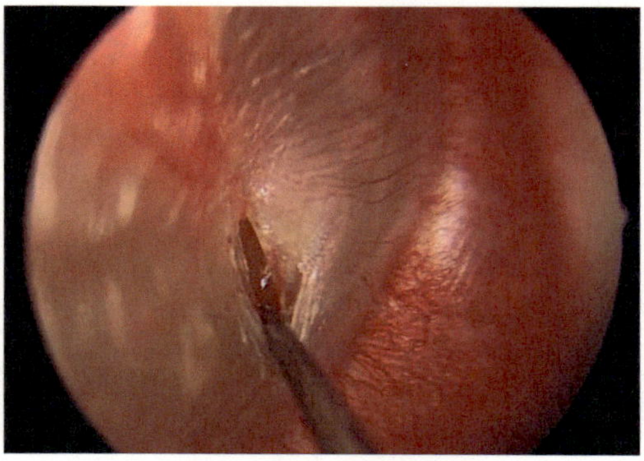

Figure 2.
Myringotomy in OME.

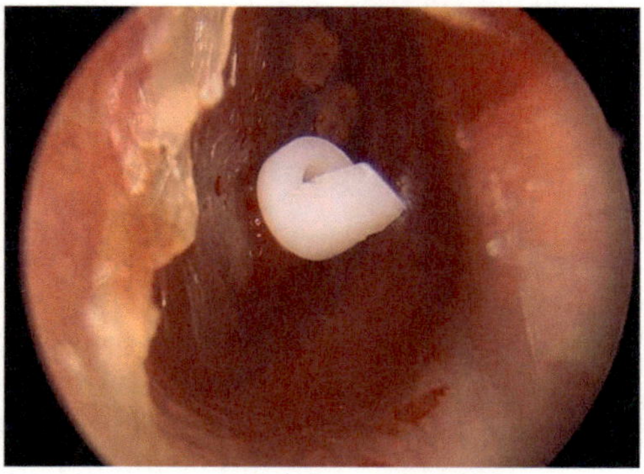

Figure 3.
Temporary ear tube placement.

purulent ear discharge through a persistent perforation of the tympanic membrane (chronic suppurative otitis media, CSOM) [38].

It has been demonstrated that the bacterial biofilm was more frequently polymicrobial near the Eustachian tube orifice [30] and it has been hypothesized its potential role as a source of otopathogens, capable of migrating and colonizing middle ear mucosa through an impaired Eustachian tube [31]. Furthermore, it has been evidenced that nasopharyngeal biofilm-producing otopathogens is more frequently represented in the nasopharynxes of young children with RAOM without chronic adenoiditis, suggesting that nasopharyngeal biofilms are independently involved in the development of recurrent middle ear infections, regardless of the presence of adenoidal hypertrophy [28].

4. Diagnosis

There are currently no universal indications for the diagnosis of chronic adenoiditis. Historically, the two instruments used for diagnostic purposes were the posterior rhinoscopy (with laryngeal mirror) and nasopharyngeal radiological examination.

Lateral X-ray imaging and local computed tomography scanning can show increased adenoid size with the possible obstruction of the upper airway [6]. However, the lack of correlation between the level of obstruction evidenced by X-ray and nasal symptoms has been demonstrated [23]. Moreover, the radiological risk from X-ray exposure should not be underestimated in children [39].

Nowadays, nasal endoscopy is considered the gold standard for diagnosis of the disease. In particular, the flexible fiber-optic scop is widely used in children, allowing a better examination of the nasal cavities and nasopharynx [2].

Many classifications have been proposed for adenoid hypertrophy, but the most relevant for the degree of obstruction of the nasopharynx is that of Parikh et al. [40]: grade 1 for adenoid tissue not in contact with adjacent structures; grade 2 for adenoid tissue in contact with the torus tubarius; grade 3 for adenoid tissue in contact with the vomer; grade 4 for adenoid tissue in contact with the soft palate.

Children typically complain of foreign body sensations at the pharynx, adhesion of the sputum, and postnasal dripping. Endoscopic examination can show mucosal edema on the surface of adenoids with the presence of different degrees of mucus or pus adhesion, while physical examination can evidence retropharyngeal folliculitis and cobblestone-like changes, the adhesion of mucinous, or purulent secretion. Other symptoms may be associated with chronic adenoiditis, such as nasal obstruction, running nose, sneezing, dry throat, and headache [6].

5. Therapeutic approaches: non-surgical therapy

The use of intranasal steroids (INS) is well known for reducing adenoid size and symptoms and it is most often the first line of treatment. A metanalysis by Alisha Chohan et al. [41] in 2015 evaluated the role of mometasone in children with adenoidal hypertrophy. Mometasone caused improvements in outcomes of nasal obstruction, snoring, total nasal symptoms, pure tone audiometry, otitis media with effusion, and quality of life. The doses used range from 100 to 400 mg, for a duration of treatment between 4 and 9 weeks. The effect of mometasone on different outcomes appeared at 6 weeks and remained till 12 weeks.

Other intranasal steroids, such as Fluticasone propionate, Beclomethasone dipropionate, and Flunisolide, are associated with improved nasal obstruction, mouth breathing, apnea, and adenoid size, reducing the rate of surgery for adenoid hypertrophy, especially in children with allergic rhinitis. Proposed mechanisms for the INS activity in adenoid hypertrophy include direct lympholytic action, inhibition of inflammation, and alteration of adenoidal bacterial flora [42].

Leukotriene inhibitors (such as Montelukast, Zafirlukast, and Pranlukast) have been proposed as non-surgical therapy for adenoidal hypertrophy. Montelukast, an oral cysteinyl leukotriene receptor antagonist indicated as preventive therapy for the inflammatory component of asthma and allergic rhinitis, has been shown to cause a reduction of adenoid size in 76% of patients [43].

A 2021 review by Ji et al. [44] on the effect of antileukotrienes on children with obstructive sleep apnea evidenced that leukotriene inhibitors improve sleep disorders and the quality of life in children with mild-to-moderate OSA, alone and in addition to intranasal steroids, reducing tonsillar and adenoid size. Side effects such as headache, nausea, and vomiting were reported only in one study.

Systemic or local antibacterial treatments are effective for chronic adenoiditis induced by bacterial infection [6], but not sufficient modes of treatment for adenoid hypertrophy. Additionally, many viruses are often associated with adenoid hypertrophy [45].

6. Therapeutic approaches: surgical therapy

Adenoidectomy with or without tonsillectomy is one of the most common ENT procedures performed in the pediatric population. The most common indication for this procedure is obstructive sleep-disordered breathing and obstructive sleep apnea syndrome (OSAS). Other indications include chronic or recurrent otitis media with effusion, chronic rhinorrhea, nasal obstruction, sinusitis, and chronic adenoiditis. The AAO-HNS 2021 guidelines for adenoidectomy are fully described in **Table 1** [46].

The traditional technique is a curettage adenoidectomy that is used by most ENT surgeons. In the last years, different surgical techniques have been proposed to reduce surgical risk and morbidity: electrocautery adenoidectomy, microdebrider adenoidectomy, and coblation adenoidectomy. The ideal technique should be quick, easy to perform, minimize postoperative pain, with a low rate of postoperative complications and relapse rate.

In the traditional adenoidectomy, the main bulk of adenoids is removed using curette or adenotome blindly (**Figure 4**), without direct visualization of the nasopharynx. Digital palpation at the end of the procedure is used by many ENT surgeons to confirm the complete removal of adenoid tissue. When the adenoids extend toward the peritubaric region or intranasally, adequate removal can be challenging, just by a blind curettage adenoidectomy [47].

In order to provide direct visualization of surgical field the use of angled mirrors and, in the last years, of endoscopes during adenoidectomy is becoming popular.

A study performed by Ark et al. [48] showed that the direct visualization of nasopharynx during adenoidectomy is necessary to fully remove the adenoid tissue. In this study, a group of patients that underwent a traditional adenoidectomy was inspected using a laryngeal mirror and only an on-fifth of them had no residual adenoid tissue. The commonest residual site was the nasopharynx roof near the choanal opening, followed by the peritubaric region.

History (One or more required)	1. Four or greater episodes of recurrent purulent rhinorrhea in prior 12 months in a child <12 years of age. One episode should be documented by intranasal examination or diagnostic imaging. 2. Persisting symptoms of adenoiditis after two courses of antibiotic therapy. One course of antibiotics should be with a B-lactamase stable antibiotic for at least 2 weeks. 3. Sleep disturbance with nasal airway obstruction persists for at least 3 months. 4. Hyponasal speech. 5. Otitis media with effusion >3 months or associated with additional sets of tubes. 6. Dental malocclusion or orofacial growth disturbance is documented by an orthodontist or dentist. 7. Cardiopulmonary complications include cor pulmonale, pulmonary hypertension, and right ventricular hypertrophy associated with upper airway obstruction. 8. Otitis media with effusion (age 4 or greater). For infectious conditions, it is recommended that documentation of infections be obtained. For hypertrophy and other noninfectious conditions documentation should include information regarding growth, weight gain, daytime performance issues such as behavior and attention, and any medical condition necessitating removal of the adenoids. Adenoid size is immaterial when the indication is sinusitis, adenoiditis, or otitis media with effusion. Allergic symptoms should have been treated with an adequate trial of allergy therapy before evaluation for non-infectious conditions.
Physical Examination (required)	1. Physical examination (required) 2. Description of uvula, palate, tonsils, nasal airway, and cervical lymph nodes. 3. Evaluation of adenoids by mirror, palpation, nasal endoscopy, or imaging only as necessary. 4. Assessment for signs of hypernasal speech or risk factors for postop voice disturbance
Tests (If abnormality suspected by history, physical examination)	1. Coagulation and bleeding evaluation based on personal or family history 2. Radiographs (lateral neck or cephalometric) 3. Sleep tape recording (if documentation of snoring or apnea is required) 4. Polysomnography in children at high risk for respiratory compromise

Table 1.
AAO-HNS 2021 guidelines for adenoidectomy.

A study by Ezzat et al. [49] performed in a cohort of 300 patients reported that an endoscopic examination after a curettage adenoidectomy showed residual adenoid tissue that required to be removed in 14.5% of cases. In this case, percentage of revision adenoidectomy after 2 years was only 0.85%. Patients that did not undergo an endoscopic examination after the procedure had a revision rate adenoidectomy of 5.6%, showing that the use of an endoscope significantly reduces the incidence of recurrence and the need for revision surgery.

In the '90s, the advent of endoscopic sinus surgery (ESS) popularized the use of intranasal endoscopes and endoscopic adenoidectomy becoming popular, permitting direct visualization of the surgical field and better removal of the adenoid tissue, mostly from the superior part of the nasopharynx and peritubal region [50].

Cannon et al. [50] called the Endoscopic Assisted Adenoidectomy (EAA) a "natural progression of endoscopic technology to allow a more complete adenoidectomy." Intranasal or transoral endoscopes can be used following traditional adenoidectomy, or in combining techniques with curettes, suction diathermy, microdebriders, and coblator [2].

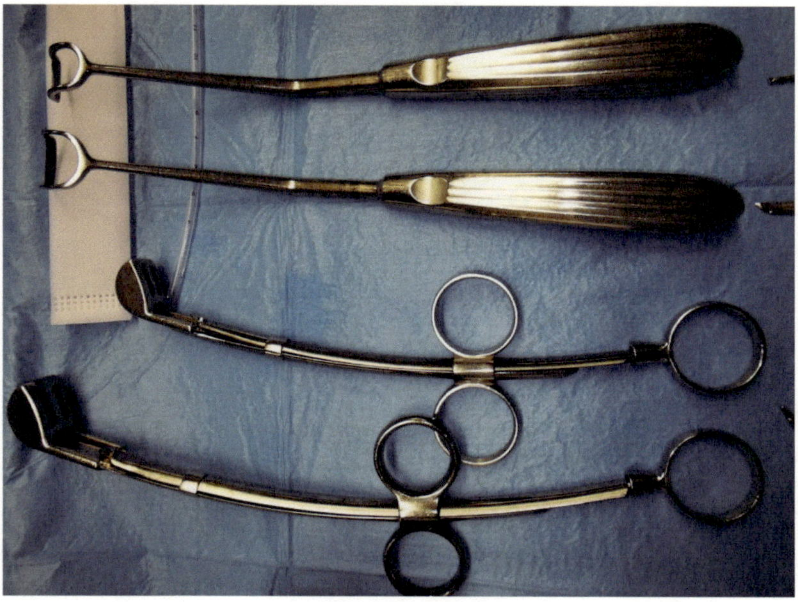

Figure 4.
Two different-sized Shambaugh adenotomes and adenoid curettes.

A Network Meta-analysis performed in 2023 by Ya-Lei Sun et al. [51] compared four approaches available for adenoidectomy (curettage adenoidectomy, suction diathermy adenoidectomy, powered vacuum shaver adenoidectomy, and plasma field ablation adenoidectomy). It evidenced that there were no significant differences between these techniques for operative time, intraoperative blood loss, and incidence of postoperative residual tissue, while plasma field ablation adenoidectomy showed lower postoperative pain scores than curettage adenoidectomy.

6.1 Traditional adenoidectomy

The traditional adenoidectomy technique includes curettes and/or adenotomes to remove the adenoidal tissue, with patient placed in the Rose position and under general anesthesia *via* oro-tracheal intubation.

The surgeon is placed at the head of the patient (**Figure 5**) and the instruments pass transorally to reach the nasopharynx and the adenoid pad, so as to remove the lymphatic nasopharyngeal tissue (**Figures 6** and 7).

The procedure is usually performed blindly, and digital palpation confirms the full removal of adenoid tissue. Following that, removal of mucus and clots is performed through nasal irrigation. After several saline irrigations, hemostasis is usually performed by placing a gauze pack in the nasopharynx for some minutes. Cold curettage potentially minimizes morbidities associated with thermal injury, but the blind procedure can theoretically damage the Eustachian tube or pharyngeal muscles and leaves residual tissue, especially in peritubaric and superior nasopharyngeal region [47].

The traditional adenoidectomy can be performed using a laryngeal mirror or an endoscope. The latter can be used following a curettage adenoidectomy to remove residual adenoid tissue transnasally with Blakesley forceps [52] or curette [53].

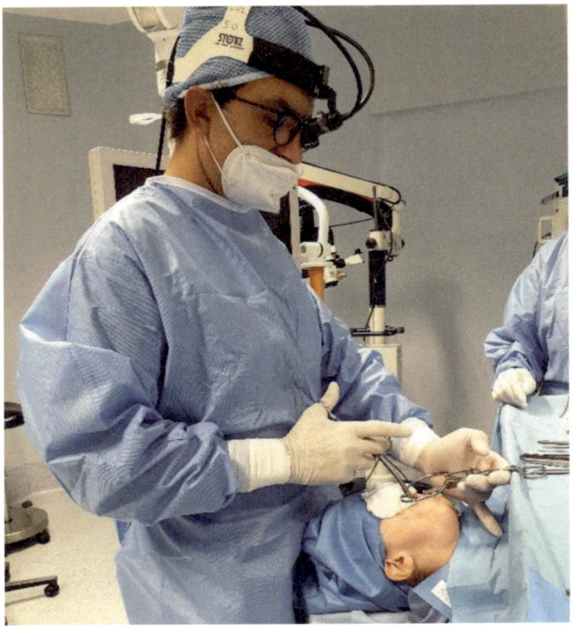

Figure 5.
Surgical position during a traditional adenoidectomy.

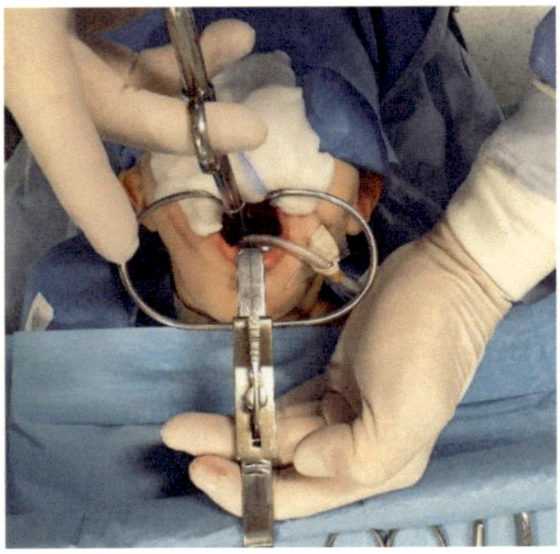

Figure 6.
External view of a traditional adenoidectomy performed with a Shambaugh adenotome.

Alternatively, the curettage adenoidectomy can be performed directly under an endoscopic guide, transnasally [54] (**Figure 8**) or transorally [55]. The advantage of these methods is the direct visualization of surgical field that would decrease the rate of residual adenoids and potential injury of the Eustachian tube (**Figure 9**).

6.2 Suction cautery adenoidectomy

In the 1980s, the use of suction electrocautery to control bleeding during curettage adenoidectomy became popular. Subsequently, suction diathermy ablation of the adenoids become a popular alternative to traditional adenoidectomy, resulting being

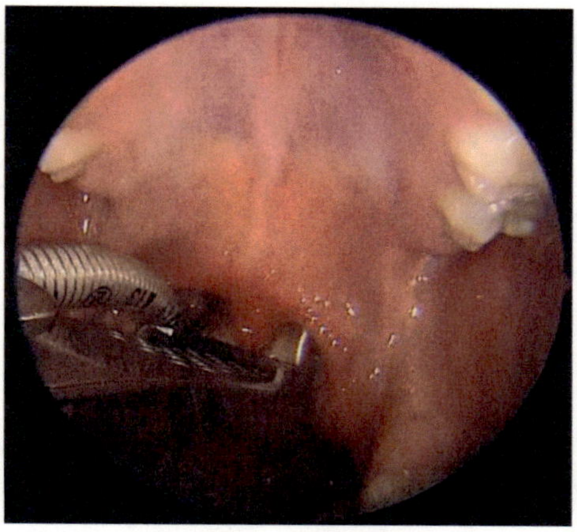

Figure 7.
Internal view of a traditional adenoidectomy performed with a Shambaugh. In the first place the tonsillar tissue adenotome.

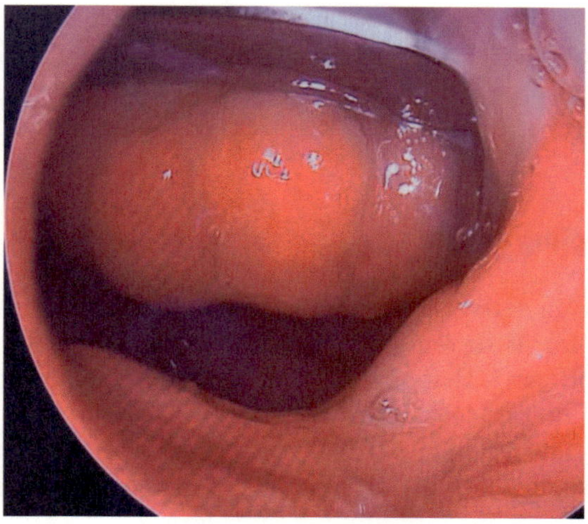

Figure 8.
Curette adenoidectomy under endoscopic vision.

the most common surgical method, as referred to in a 2007 survey among the members of the American Society of Pediatric Otolaryngology [56]. The most common advantage according to this technique is the lower intra-operative bleeding loss and the ability to precisely remove adenoid tissue in the choanal region.

The procedure is done under general endotracheal anesthesia and the adenoid plate is visualized indirectly through a mirror placed in the oropharynx or a transoral angled endoscope. Diathermy ablation of the adenoid pad is performed using an insulated, curved Frazier-type suction system, and a monopolar is applied to the non-insulated portion of the suction or suction coagulator. The suction electrocautery device is applied to the adenoid pad starting from the superior part. The adenoidal tissue shrinks, as the suction device evacuates the smoke. The procedure is completed when the choanae are clearly visible and the nasopharynx presents a smooth level contour. It is important not to traumatize soft palate, Eustachian tube, or pharyngeal wall, so as to avoid scarring and nasopharyngeal stenosis [57].

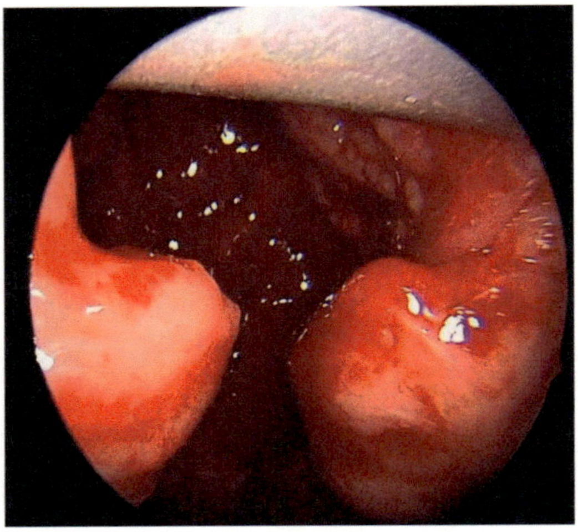

Figure 9.
Transoral endoscopic view after traditional adenoidectomy.

A 2009 meta-analysis by Reed et al. [58] demonstrates that suction cautery adenoidectomy has a significantly lower rate of intra-operative hemorrhage and decreases operative time compared to the curette adenoidectomy keeping equivalent short-term outcomes.

6.3 Coblation adenoidectomy

The word Coblation derives from "Controlled Ablation." Intended as a low-thermal technology for tissue removal, it recently became popular in ENT procedures. The principle of coblation is that of producing a plasma field using radiofrequency through an electrically conductive fluid, like isotonic sodium chloride solution, so as to remove tissue at a low temperature (40–70°C). Other procedures based on electrosurgical devices such as electrocautery adenoidectomy reach temperatures around 400–600°C. Coblation technology allows tissue removal with a low risk of thermal injury, creating a stable plasma layer of only 100–200 μm thickness around the active electrode, allowing precise tissue excision [59].

Endoscopic-assisted coblation adenoidectomy combines both the advantage of scope view and coblation technology. Several studies have shown that coblation adenoidectomy presents lower post-operative pain than curette adenoidectomy, reducing the use of post-operative drugs and loss of working days for parents, due to faster post-surgical healing. The concomitant use of the endoscope and the small wand tip of coblator allow selective removal of adenoid tissue reaching both the most cranial part of adenoid pad and the intranasal extension, preserving structures such as the Eustachian tube and pharyngeal mucosa. Another advantage is the ability to ablate and coagulate at the same time, as referred disadvantages are the need for a pediatric endoscopic set, the longer pre-operative set-up time, the need for a learning curve in pediatric endoscopy, and the inability to perform a histopathological examination [51, 59–61].

In a study conducted by Bidaye et al. [59] comparing curette adenoidectomy and endoscopic assisted coblation adenoidectomy, it was seen that the percentage of adenoid remnant is 40% with the traditional technique, while it was 0% with the coblator, with significantly lower postoperative pain in the coblation group. The same results were observed in Hapalia et al.'s [60] and Di Rienzo Businco et al.'s [61] comparative studies, between endoscopic coblation technique and cold curettage adenoidectomy, showing a lower residual adenoid rate and postoperative pain with the former technique.

6.4 Microdebrider adenoidectomy

Power-assisted instruments, such as microdebriders, were first used in endoscopic sinus surgery to treat inflammatory diseases and became popular in adenoidectomy in the last years. The adenoid pad can be removed under laryngeal mirror or under an endoscopic vision, thus permitting a better view of the field. Endoscopes can be used transanally (0° scope) or transorally (45° or 70° scopes). The first adenoidectomy with power-assisted instruments performed under transnasal endoscopic view was first reported by Yanagisawa in 1997 [62].

Costantini et al. [63] proposed a trans-oral adenoidectomy using 40° curved microdebriders and 70° scopes. The instrument is introduced through the mouth and the smooth tip of the microdebrider is placed into the recess between the side vegetations and the tubaric ostium to remove the adenoid pad without damaging the Eustachian tube. At the end of resection, a gauze packing is transorally placed in the nasopharynx to perform adequate hemostasis. This procedure offers an improved visual field and extreme precision in removing the adenoid tissue. Compared with the adenotome or curette removal, it permits to remove adenoid tissue in the most important sites: the choanal and tubaric regions. The continuous suction of the microdebrider during the resection permits for maintenance of a bloodless field, and thus, post-operative bleeding loss is extremely low, comparable with adenoidectomy techniques [51].

In transnasal power-assisted adenoidectomy with transansal endoscopic control [64], both instruments pass through the nostril (**Figures 10** and **11**). Under endoscopic vision, the shaver cannula is passed into the nose with the suction switched off, so as to not damage the nasal mucosa. The adenoid pad is removed under endoscopic control with care not to lacerate the torus tubarius. Working from proximal to distal the adenoid tissue is removed under a bloodless field thanks to the continuous suctions. A small inferior rim of adenoid tissue can be left intact intentionally, thus preserving the velopharyngeal sphincter.

However, in the presence of a bulky adenoid pad, a pure microdebrider adenoidectomy is time consuming. One possibility is to perform the first step with standard adenoid instruments (curette and adenotome) and then enable microdebriders to remove, if needed, the residual adenoid tissue under a transnsal endoscopic view [65].

Sometimes, the use of transnasal microdebrider under transnasal endoscopic view can be difficult, especially in younger children. The insertion through the nose of both instruments is challenging and the maneuverability is limited. The Transoral Endonasal-Controlled Combined Adenoidectomy (TECCA) technique [66] permits better maneuverability of the instruments in case of narrow nasal spaces and a complete clearance of nasopharyngeal area. As a first step, a traditional transoral adenoidectomy is performed. After that, the residual adenoid is checked with transnasal endoscopy with 0° rigid fiber optic. If residual adenoid tissue is still present, it gets fully removed with curved microdebriders (**Figure 12**).

This procedure carries no additional risk compared to other techniques and is effective to remove the peritubaric and superior adenoidal tissue without damaging the surrounding structures [67].

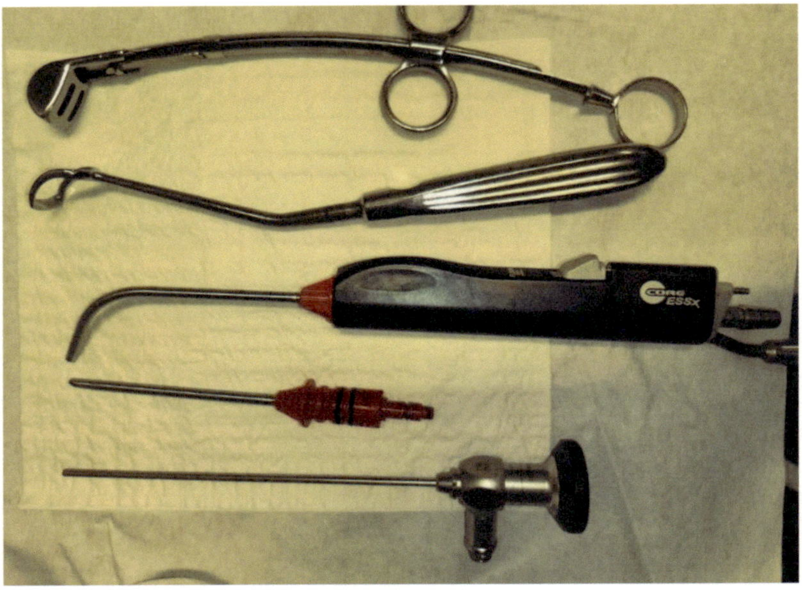

Figure 10.
Endoscope (0°), curved and straight microdebriders, curette, and Shambaugh adenotome.

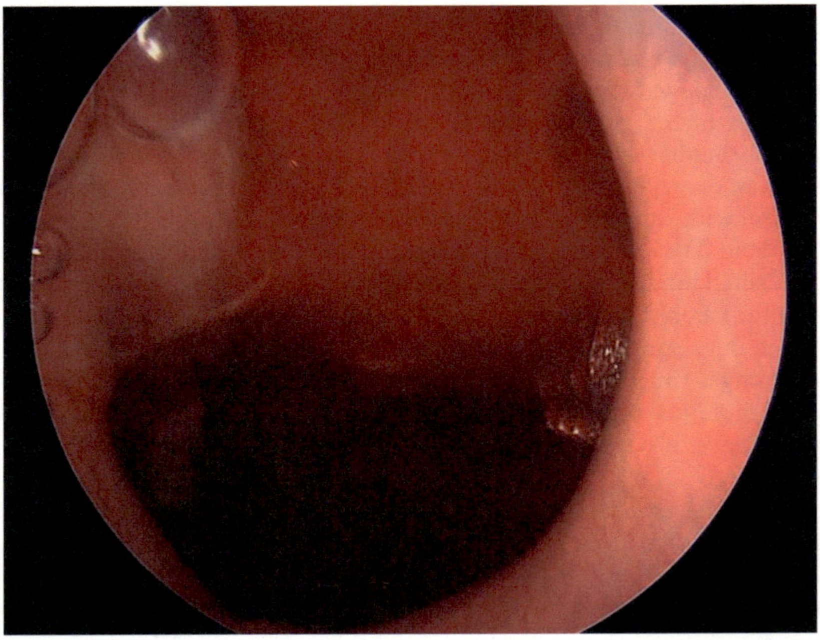

Figure 11.
Transnasal power-assisted adenoidectomy with transansal endoscopic control adenotome.

Endoscopic power-assisted adenoidectomy is a safe procedure, with minimal intra-operative and post-operative bleeding loss, low post-operative pain, and faster recovery. The endoscopic view gives greater control of the surgical field allowing a complete clearance of adenoid tissue [68].

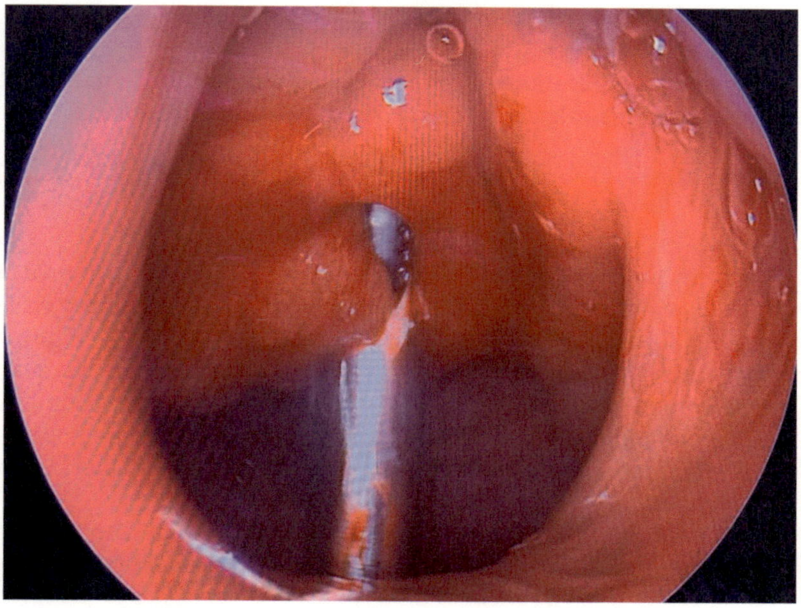

Figure 12.
TECCA technique.

7. Adenoidectomy complication

Adenoidectomy in children is generally a safe procedure with a low rate of complications. The most frequent is hemorrhage, distinct in primary (within 24 hours following surgery) and secondary (after 24 hours following surgery). The rate of the former is between 0.5 and 0.8%, while the latter is very low. The risk of bleeding is additive if a tonsillectomy is associated with the procedure [69, 70].

Velopharyngeal insufficiency (VPI) is a rare but well-recognized complication of adenoidectomy with an impact on the communication skills of a child. It occurs when an inadequate velopharyngeal closure is achieved during speech and/or swallowing, with hypernasal voice quality, nasal regurgitation, and poor speech output. VPI following adenoidectomy is usually transient and should resolve in 3–6 months. Patients with cleft palate, bifid uvula, poor palatal motion, and deep pharynx have a higher risk of developing VPI and should undergo a partial superior adenoidectomy so as to decrease risk. Above 50% of patients with VPI will respond to speech therapy and, in the case of treatment failure, various surgical options are available [71].

Grisel syndrome or non-traumatic atlantoaxial rotary subluxation is a rare adenoidectomy complication, with an increased rate in Down syndrome children. Clinical symptoms are torticollis, pain during neck rotations, and fever. Radiograms and CT scans of the cervical spine are required to confirm the diagnosis. Surgical treatment is indicated in case of high-grade instability or failure of conservative treatment [72].

Nasopharyngeal stenosis is the interruption of the normal communication between nasopharynx and oropharynx, due to the fusion of tonsillar pillars and soft palate to the oropharyngeal posterior wall, creating a strong fibrous wall. It is a rare complication that occurs in excessive electrocautery and dissection.

Its management is surgical: Bilateral Z-pharyngoplasty and palatal eversion are the treatment of choice [73].

Other, very rare, complications described in the literature, are vertebral osteomyelitis, cerebrospinal fluid leakage, and temporomandibular joint dysfunction [45].

8. Conclusions

Adenoidectomy is one of the most common ENT procedures. Traditional curettage adenoidectomy is widely used and it is performed blindly, without direct visualization of the surgical field. In the last years, several other techniques have been proposed: electrocautery adenoidectomy, microdebrider adenoidectomy, and coblation adenoidectomy, with a low rate of residual adenoid tissue and post-operative complications. "Blind" curettage adenoidectomy remains a procedure with good outcomes, but it can fail in obtaining full removal of adenoid pad, especially in the peritubaric, superior, and choanal regions.

Combination of one of the previous surgical techniques along with the direct visualization of the surgical field with endoscopes (transnasally or transorally), allows complete removal of the adenoid tissue and avoids damages to the surrounding structures.

Conflict of interest

The authors declare no conflict of interest.

Author details

Georgios Giourgos[1*], Alberto Luchena[2] and Chiara Bovi[3]

1 Department of Neurosciences, Section of Otorhinolaryngology and Skull Base Microsurgery, Bergamo, Italy

2 Department of Otorhinolaryngology, University of Pavia, Foundation IRCCS Policlinico San Matteo, Pavia, Italy

3 Otolaryngology Department, Azienda Ospedaliera Universitaria Senese, Siena, Italy

*Address all correspondence to: ggdoc1@yahoo.com

References

[1] Bowers I, Shermetaro C. Adenoiditis. [Updated 2022 Nov 22]. In: StatPearls [Internet]. Treasure Island (FL): StatPearls Publishing; 2022 Available from: https://www.ncbi.nlm.nih.gov/books/NBK536931/

[2] Brambilla I, Pusateri A, Pagella F, Caimmi D, Caimmi S, Licari A, et al. Adenoids in children: Advances in immunology, diagnosis, and surgery. Clinical Anatomy. 2014;**27**(3):346-352. DOI: 10.1002/ca.22373 Epub 2014 Feb 18

[3] Cummings W, Charles S. Text Book of Otolaryngology. 5th ed. Elsevier, Vol. 32010. Chapter 181

[4] Spector S, Bautista AG. Respiratory obstruction caused by acute tonsillitis and acute adenoiditis. New York State Journal of Medicine. 1956;**56**(13):2118-2119

[5] Karpova EP, Kharina DV. Vozmozhnosti ratsional'noi farmakoterapii adenoidita u detei [The possibilities for the rational pharmacotherapy of adenoiditis in the children]. Vestn Otorinolaringologii. 2016;**81**(5):73-76. Russian. DOI: 10.17116/otorino201681573-76

[6] Wang H. Chronic adenoiditis. The Journal of International Medical Research.2020;**48**(11):300060520971458. DOI: 10.1177/0300060520971458

[7] Günel C, Kırdar S, Ömürlü İK, Ağdaş F. Detection of the Epstein-Barr virus, human bocavirus and novel KI and KU polyomaviruses in adenotonsillar tissues. International Journal of Pediatric Otorhinolaryngology. 2015;**79**(3):423-427. DOI: 10.1016/j.ijporl.2015.01.007 Epub 2015 Jan 15

[8] Elwany S, Ibrahim AA, Mandour Z, Talaat I. Effect of passive smoking on the ultrastructure of the nasal mucosa in children. The Laryngoscope. 2012;**122**(5):965-969. DOI: 10.1002/lary.23246 Epub 2012 Mar 23

[9] Marseglia GL, Avanzini MA, Caimmi S, Caimmi D, Marseglia A, Valsecchi C, et al. Passive exposure to smoke results in defective interferon-gamma production by adenoids in children with recurrent respiratory infections. Journal of Interferon & Cytokine Research. 2009;**29**(8):427-432. DOI: 10.1089/jir.2008.0108

[10] Shin JH, Kim BG, Kim BY, Kim SW, Kim SW, Kim H. Is there an association between vitamin D deficiency and adenotonsillar hypertrophy in children with sleep-disordered breathing? BMC Pediatrics. 2018;**18**(1):196. DOI: 10.1186/s12887-018-1178-8

[11] Sadeghi-Shabestari M, Jabbari Moghaddam Y, Ghaharri H. Is there any correlation between allergy and adenotonsillar tissue hypertrophy? International Journal of Pediatric Otorhinolaryngology. 2011;**75**(4):589-591. DOI: 10.1016/j.ijporl.2011.01.026 Epub 2011 Mar 5

[12] Modrzynski M, Zawisza E. An analysis of the incidence of adenoid hypertrophy in allergic children. International Journal of Pediatric Otorhinolaryngology. 2007;**71**(5):713-719. DOI: 10.1016/j.ijporl.2006.12.018 Epub 2007 Feb 5

[13] Altıntoprak N, Kar M, Bayar Muluk N, Oktemer T, Ipci K, Birdane L, et al. Update on local allergic rhinitis. International Journal of Pediatric Otorhinolaryngology. 2016;**87**:105-109.

DOI: 10.1016/j.ijporl.2016.06.008 Epub 2016 Jun 7

[14] Shin SY, Ye YM, Eun YG, Kim SW, Cho JS, Park HS. Local IgE-mediated hypersensitivity to Alternaria in pediatric adenoid tissue. International Journal of Pediatric Otorhinolaryngology. 2012;**76**(10):1423-1428. DOI: 10.1016/j.ijporl.2012.06.015 Epub 2012 Jul 6

[15] Shin SY, Choi SJ, Hur GY, Lee KH, Kim SW, Cho JS, et al. Local production of total IgE and specific antibodies to the house dust mite in adenoid tissue. Pediatric Allergy and Immunology. 2009;**20**(2):134-141. DOI: 10.1111/j.1399-3038.2008.00756.x Epub 2008 Jul 24

[16] Brandtzaeg P. Potential of nasopharynx-associated lymphoid tissue for vaccine responses in the airways. American Journal of Respiratory and Critical Care Medicine. 2011;**183**(12):1595-1604. DOI: 10.1164/rccm.201011-1783OC Epub 2011 Mar 18

[17] Cho KS, Kim SH, Hong SL, Lee J, Mun SJ, Roh YE, et al. Local atopy in childhood adenotonsillar hypertrophy. American Journal of Rhinology & Allergy. 2018;**32**(3):160-166. DOI: 10.1177/1945892418765003 Epub 2018 Apr 12

[18] Zhang X, Sun B, Li S, Jin H, Zhong N, Zeng G. Local atopy is more relevant than serum sIgE in reflecting allergy in childhood adenotonsillar hypertrophy. Pediatric Allergy and Immunology. 2013;**24**:422-426

[19] Costa EC Jr, Sabino HA, Miura CS, Azevedo CB, Menezes UP, Valera FC, et al. Atopy and adenotonsillar hypertrophy in mouth breathers from a reference center. Brazilian Journal of Otorhinolaryngology. 2013;**79**(6):663-667. DOI: 10.5935/1808-8694.20130123

[20] Carr E, Obholzer R, Caulfield H. A prospective study to determine the incidence of atopy in children undergoing adenotonsillectomy for obstructive sleep apnea. International Journal of Pediatric Otorhinolaryngology. 2007;**71**(1):19-22. DOI: 10.1016/j.ijporl.2006.08.011 Epub 2006 Sep 18

[21] Griffin JL, Ramadan HH, Adham RE. Prevalence of IgE-mediated hypersensitivity in children with adenotonsillar disease. Archives of Otolaryngology–Head & Neck Surgery. 1994;**120**(2):150-153. DOI: 10.1001/archotol.1994.01880260022005

[22] Alexopoulos EI, Bizakis J, Gourgoulianis K, Kaditis AG. Atopy does not affect the frequency of adenotonsillar hypertrophy and sleep apnoea in children who snore. Acta Paediatrica. 2014;**103**(12):1239-1243. DOI: 10.1111/apa.12774 Epub 2014 Sep 28

[23] Cassano P, Gelardi M, Cassano M, Fiorella ML, Fiorella R. Adenoid tissue rhinopharyngeal obstruction grading based on fiberendoscopic findings: A novel approach to therapeutic management. International Journal of Pediatric Otorhinolaryngology. 2003;**67**(12):1303-1309. DOI: 10.1016/j.ijporl.2003.07.018

[24] Zuliani G, Carron M, Gurrola J, Coleman C, Haupert M, Berk R, et al. Identification of adenoid biofilms in chronic rhinosinusitis. International Journal of Pediatric Otorhinolaryngology. 2006;**70**(9):1613-1617. DOI: 10.1016/j.ijporl.2006.05.002 Epub 2006 Jun 16

[25] Kania R, Vironneau P, Dang H, Bercot B, Cambau E, Verillaud B, et al. Bacterial biofilm in adenoids of children with chronic otitis media. Part I: A case control study of prevalence of biofilms in adenoids, risk factors

and middle ear biofilms. Acta Otolaryngologica. 2019;**139**(4):345-350. DOI: 10.1080/00016489.2019.1571282 Epub 2019 Feb 26

[26] Torretta S, Drago L, Marchisio P, Mattina R, Clemente IA, Pignataro L. Diagnostic accuracy of nasopharyngeal swabs in detecting biofilm-producing bacteria in chronic adenoiditis: A preliminary study. Otolaryngology–Head and Neck Surgery. 2011;**144**(5):784-788. DOI: 10.1177/0194599810394955

[27] Torretta S, Drago L, Marchisio P, Gaffuri M, Clemente IA, Pignataro L. Topographic distribution of biofilm-producing bacteria in adenoid subsites of children with chronic or recurrent middle ear infections. The Annals of Otology, Rhinology, and Laryngology. 2013;**122**(2):109-113. DOI: 10.1177/000348941312200206

[28] Torretta S, Marchisio P, Drago L, Baggi E, De Vecchi E, Garavello W, et al. Nasopharyngeal biofilm-producing otopathogens in children with nonsevere recurrent acute otitis media. Otolaryngology–Head and Neck Surgery. 2012;**146**(6):991-996. DOI: 10.1177/0194599812438169 Epub 2012 Feb 21

[29] Nazzari E, Torretta S, Pignataro L, Marchisio P, Esposito S. Role of biofilm in children with recurrent upper respiratory tract infections. European Journal of Clinical Microbiology & Infectious Diseases. 2015;**34**(3):421-429. DOI: 10.1007/s10096-014-2261-1 Epub 2014 Oct 16

[30] Drago L, Cappelletti L, De Vecchi E, Pignataro L, Torretta S, Mattina R. Antiadhesive and antibiofilm activity of hyaluronic acid against bacteria responsible for respiratory tract infections. APMIS. 2014;**122**(10):1013-1019. DOI: 10.1111/apm.12254 Epub 2014 Apr 4

[31] Torretta S, Drago L, Marchisio P, Ibba T, Pignataro L. Role of biofilms in children with chronic adenoiditis and middle ear disease. Journal of Clinical Medicine. 2019;**8**(5):671. DOI: 10.3390/jcm8050671

[32] Marzouk H, Aynehchi B, Thakkar P, Abramowitz T, Goldsmith A. The utility of nasopharyngeal culture in the management of chronic adenoiditis. International Journal of Pediatric Otorhinolaryngology. 2012;**76**(10):1413-1415. DOI: 10.1016/j.ijporl.2012.06.012 Epub 2012 Jul 9

[33] Fernández Cornejo VJ, Martínez-Lage JF, Piqueras C, Gelabert A, Poza M. Inflammatory atlanto-axial subluxation (Grisel's syndrome) in children: Clinical diagnosis and management. Child's Nervous System. 2003;**19**(5-6):342-347. DOI: 10.1007/s00381-003-0749-6 Epub 2003 Jun 3

[34] Tomonaga K, Kurono Y, Chaen T, Mogi G. Adenoids and otitis media with effusion: Nasopharyngeal flora. American Journal of Otolaryngology. 1989;**10**(3):204-207. DOI: 10.1016/0196-0709(89)90064-1

[35] Kocyigit M, Ortekin SG, Cakabay T, Ozkaya G, Bezgin SU, Adali MK. Frequency of serous otitis media in children without otolaryngological symptoms. International Archives of Otorhinolaryngology. 2017;**21**(2):161-164. DOI: 10.1055/s-0036-1584362 Epub 2016 Jun 3

[36] American Academy of Family Physicians, American Academy of Otolaryngology-Head and Neck Surgery, American Academy of Pediatrics Subcommittee on Otitis Media With Effusion. Otitis media with effusion.

Pediatrics. 2004;**113**(5):1412-1429. DOI: 10.1542/peds.113.5.1412

[37] Gates GA, Klein JO, Lim DJ, Mogi G, Ogra PL, Pararella MM, et al. Recent advances in otitis media. 1. Definitions, terminology, and classification of otitis media. The Annals of Otology, Rhinology & Laryngology. Supplement. 2002;**188**:8-18. DOI: 10.1177/00034894021110s304

[38] Jensen RG, Koch A, Homøe P. The risk of hearing loss in a population with a high prevalence of chronic suppurative otitis media. International Journal of Pediatric Otorhinolaryngology. 2013;**77**(9):1530-1535. DOI: 10.1016/j.ijporl.2013.06.025 Epub 2013 Jul 29

[39] Cho JH, Lee DH, Lee NS, Won YS, Yoon HR, Suh BD. Size assessment of adenoid and nasopharyngeal airway by acoustic rhinometry in children. The Journal of Laryngology and Otology. 1999;**113**(10):899-905. DOI: 10.1017/s0022215100145530

[40] Parikh SR, Coronel M, Lee JJ, Brown SM. Validation of a new grading system for endoscopic examination of adenoid hypertrophy. Otolaryngology - Head and Neck Surgery. 2006;**135**(5): 684-687. DOI: 10.1016/j.otohns.2006.05.003

[41] Chohan A, Lal A, Chohan K, Chakravarti A, Gomber S. Systematic review and meta-analysis of randomized controlled trials on the role of mometasone in adenoid hypertrophy in children. International Journal of Pediatric Otorhinolaryngology. 2015;**79**(10):1599-1608. DOI: 10.1016/j.ijporl.2015.07.009

[42] Scadding G. Non-surgical treatment of adenoidal hypertrophy: The role of treating IgE-mediated inflammation. Pediatric Allergy and Immunology. 2010;**21**(8):1095-1106. DOI: 10.1111/j.1399-3038.2010.01012.x

[43] Shokouhi F, Meymaneh Jahromi A, Majidi MR, Salehi M. Montelukast in adenoid hypertrophy: Its effect on size and symptoms. Iranian Journal of Otorhinolaryngology. 2015;**27**(83):443-448

[44] Ji T, Lu T, Qiu Y, et al. The efficacy and safety of montelukast in children with obstructive sleep apnea: A systematic review and meta-analysis. Sleep Medicine. 2021;**78**:193-201. DOI: 10.1016/j.sleep.2020.11.009

[45] Schupper AJ, Nation J, Pransky S. Adenoidectomy in children: What is the evidence and what is its role? Current Otorhinolaryngology Reports. 2018;**6**(1):64-73. DOI: 10.1007/s40136-018-0190-8

[46] AAO-HNS. Clinical Indicators: Adenoidectomy [Internet]. 2021. Available from: https://www.entnet.org/resource/clinical-indicators-adenoidectomy/

[47] Buchinsky FJ, Lowry MA, Isaacson G. Do adenoids regrow after excision? Otolaryngology–Head and Neck Surgery. 2000;**123**(5):576-581. DOI: 10.1067/mhn.2000.110727

[48] Ark N, Kurtaran H, Ugur KS, Yilmaz T, Ozboduroglu AA, Mutlu C. Comparison of adenoidectomy methods: Examining with digital palpation vs. visualizing the placement of the curette. International Journal of Pediatric Otorhinolaryngology. 2010;**74**(6):649-651. DOI: 10.1016/j.ijporl.2010.03.012

[49] Ezzat WF. Role of endoscopic nasal examination in reduction of nasopharyngeal adenoid recurrence rates. International Journal of Pediatric Otorhinolaryngology.

2010;**74**(4):404-406. DOI: 10.1016/j.ijporl.2010.01.016

[50] Cannon CR, Replogle WH, Schenk MP. Endoscopic-assisted adenoidectomy. Otolaryngology–Head and Neck Surgery. 1999;**121**(6):740-744. DOI: 10.1053/hn.1999.v121.a98201

[51] Sun YL, Yuan B, Kong F. Comparison between different approaches applied in pediatric adenoidectomy: A network meta-analysis. The Annals of Otology, Rhinology, and Laryngology. 2023;**132**(2):207-216. DOI: 10.1177/00034894221081612

[52] Huang HM, Chao MC, Chen YL, Hsiao HR. A combined method of conventional and endoscopic adenoidectomy. The Laryngoscope. 1998;**108**(7):1104-1106. DOI: 10.1097/00005537-199807000-00028

[53] Regmi D, Mathur NN, Bhattarai M. Rigid endoscopic evaluation of conventional curettage adenoidectomy. The Journal of Laryngology and Otology. 2011;**125**(1):53-58. DOI: 10.1017/S0022215110002100

[54] Wan YM, Wong KC, Ma KH. Endoscopic-guided adenoidectomy using a classic adenoid curette: A simple way to improve adenoidectomy. Hong Kong Medical Journal. 2005;**11**(1):42-44

[55] El-Badrawy A, Abdel-Aziz M. Transoral endoscopic adenoidectomy. International Journal of Otolaryngology. 2009;**2009**:949315. DOI: 10.1155/2009/949315

[56] Skilbeck CJ, Tweedie DJ, Lloyd-Thomas AR, Albert DM. Suction diathermy for adenoidectomy: Complications and risk of recurrence. International Journal of Pediatric Otorhinolaryngology. 2007;**71**(6):917-920. DOI: 10.1016/j.ijporl.2007.03.001

[57] Elluru RG, Johnson L, Myer CM 3rd. Electrocautery adenoidectomy compared with curettage and power-assisted methods. Laryngoscope. 2002;**112**(8 Pt 2 Suppl 100):23-25. DOI: 10.1002/lary.5541121409

[58] Reed J, Sridhara S, Brietzke SE. Electrocautery adenoidectomy outcomes: A meta-analysis. Otolaryngology - Head and Neck Surgery. 2009;**140**(2):148-153. DOI 10.1016/j.otohns.2008.11.030

[59] Bidaye R, Vaid N, Desarda K. Comparative analysis of conventional cold curettage versus endoscopic assisted coblation adenoidectomy. The Journal of Laryngology and Otology. 2019;**133**(4):294-299. DOI: 10.1017/S0022215119000227

[60] Hapalia VB, Panchal AJ, Kumar R, et al. Pediatric adenoidectomy: A comparative study between cold curettage and coblation technique. Indian Journal of Otolaryngology and Head & Neck Surgery. 2022;**74**(Suppl. 2):1163-1168. DOI: 10.1007/s12070-020-02247-4

[61] Di Rienzo BL, Angelone AM, Mattei A, Ventura L, Lauriello M. Paediatric adenoidectomy: Endoscopic coblation technique compared to cold curettage. Acta Otorhinolaryngologica Italica. 2012;**32**(2):124-129

[62] Yanagisawa E, Weaver EM. Endoscopic adenoidectomy with the microdebrider. Ear, Nose & Throat Journal. 1997;**76**(2):72-74

[63] Costantini F, Salamanca F, Amaina T, Zibordi F. Videoendoscopic adenoidectomy with microdebrider. Acta Otorhinolaryngologica Italica. 2008;**28**(1):26-29

[64] Al-Mazrou KA, Al-Qahtani A, Al-Fayez AI. Effectiveness of transnasal endoscopic powered adenoidectomy in patients with choanal adenoids. International Journal of Pediatric Otorhinolaryngology. 2009;**73**(12):1650-1652. DOI: 10.1016/j.ijporl.2009.08.019

[65] Pagella F, Pusateri A, Giourgos G, Matti E. Evolution of the adenoidectomy in the endoscopic era. Advances in Endoscopic Surgery. Ed Intechopen; 2011:131-154. DOI: 10.5772/23177

[66] Pagella F, Pusateri A, Matti E, Giourgos G. Transoral endonasal-controlled combined adenoidectomy (TECCA). The Laryngoscope. 2010;**120**(10):2008-2010. DOI: 10.1002/lary.21070

[67] Pagella F, Pusateri A, Canzi P, et al. The evolution of the adenoidectomy: Analysis of different power-assisted techniques. International Journal of Immunopathology and Pharmacology. 2011;**24**(4 Suppl):55-59. DOI: 10.1177/03946320110240S411

[68] Wadhera R, Vashist A, Kumar P, Ghai A. Endoscopic adenoidectomy with microdebrider. Indian Journal of Otolaryngology and Head and Neck Surgery. 2022;**74**(Suppl 2):1314-1318. DOI: 10.1007/s12070-021-02416-z

[69] Tomkinson A, Harrison W, Owens D, Fishpool S, Temple M. Postoperative hemorrhage following adenoidectomy. The Laryngoscope. 2012;**122**(6):1246-1253. DOI: 10.1002/lary.23279

[70] Lowe D, Brown P, Yung M. Adenoidectomy technique in the United Kingdom and postoperative hemorrhage. Otolaryngology–Head and Neck Surgery. 2011;**145**(2):314-318. DOI: 10.1177/0194599811403119

[71] Lambert EM, You P, Kacmarynski DS, Rosenberg TL. Adenoidectomy and persistent velopharyngeal insufficiency: Considerations, risk factors, and treatment. International Journal of Pediatric Otorhinolaryngology. 2021;**149**:110846. DOI: 10.1016/j.ijporl.2021.110846

[72] Pini N, Ceccoli M, Bergonzini P, Iughetti L. Grisel's syndrome in children: Two case reports and systematic review of the literature. Case Reports in Pediatrics. 2020;**2020**:8819758. Published 2020 Nov 12. DOI: 10.1155/2020/8819758

[73] Abdel-Fattah G. Palatal eversion for the treatment of combined nasopharyngeal stenosis and tonsillar pillars adhesion. International Journal of Pediatric Otorhinolaryngology. 2016;**90**:227-230. DOI: 10.1016/j.ijporl.2016.09.028

Chapter 2

Peritonsillar and Intratonsillar Abscess: A Review on Clinical Features, Managements and Complications

Hardip Singh Gendeh and Balwant Singh Gendeh

Abstract

Peritonsillar and intratonsillar abscesses are one of the not too frequent emergencies encountered by the ENT fraternity. Tonsillitis refers to inflammation of the tonsils, whereas peritonsillitis refers to cellulitis with or without an abscess collection within the surrounding soft tissue of the tonsils. Peritonsillar abscess is often unilateral, while peritonsillitis may be bilateral in 20% of cases, whereas intratonsillar abscess is rare with an incidence of 7%. The shared symptoms of peritonsillitis and intratonsillar abscess include fever, trismus, deviation of uvula and referred pain. These shared symptoms have placed many physicians in a dilemma, resulting in an intratonsillar abscess to be missed. The medical therapy consists of intravenous antibiotics and intravenous fluids. A needle aspiration is useful when a diagnosis is uncertain. Aspiration of pus is diagnostic confirming a peritonsillar abscess from a peritonsillar cellulitis. Incision and drainage can be performed for intratonsillar abscess not responding to treatment or a failed needle aspiration, which is preferably performed under general anesthesia for children. Elective tonsillectomy should be indicated for patients with recurrent peritonsillar abscess. CT contrast is useful to identify complications arising mainly in retropharyngeal or parapharyngeal abscess and to know its extension, spread and drainage approaches.

Keywords: peritonsillar abscess, intratonsillar abscess, clinical presentation, complications, imaging, treatment

1. Introduction

The tonsils are oval shaped lymphoid tissues situated at the oropharynx between the anterior and posterior pillars. Its boundaries are the soft palate superiorly, base of tongue inferiorly, palatoglossal arch anteriorly and palatopharyngeous arch posteriorly. It is part of the Waldeyer's ring, named after Heinrich Wilhelm Gottfried von Waldeyer-Hartz who described the incomplete ring of lymphoid tissue within the nasopharynx and oropharynx in 1884 [1]. The ring consists of the pharyngeal tonsils (adenoids), tubal tonsils (tonsils of the torus tuberous), palatine tonsils and lingual tonsils. The earlier two are covered by stratified columnar epithelium while the latter two are lined by stratified non-keratinized squamous epithelium [1]. It is the palatine tonsils that are commonly referred to as tonsils by the lay person. Tonsils are involved in immunity as it is a form of lymphoid tissue rich in B cells that stimulates plasma cells and production of antibodies. It is most active within 4 to 10 years of age and in most individuals, undergoes involution after puberty.

Tonsillitis, peritonsillitis and intratonsillar abscess are pathology associated with inflammation of the tonsils and its surrounding soft tissues. Tonsillitis refers to inflammation of the tonsils. Peritonsillitis on the other hand refers to cellulitis with or without an abscess collection within the surrounding soft tissue (soft palate) of the tonsils. They are at different stages to the disease process, differentiated only by the presence of pus from the peritonsillar space. The peritonsillar space is essentially the loose connective tissue that separates the tonsils or its capsule which itself is part of the pharyngobasilar fascia. A peritonsillar abscess may be localized or occur within many small locules of the peritonsillar space [2]. This may cause aspiration of an abscess difficult, hence such cases are treated as a cellulitis. If abscess is evident and or drained within the peritonsillar space, then it is termed a peritonsillar abscess. Without imaging a peritonsillar abscess may be missed especially when there is no yield on aspiration or incision and drainage due to multiple small locules that are being missed. Peritonsillar abscess is often unilateral while peritonsillitis may be bilateral in 20% of cases [2].

An intratonsillar abscess occurs when the abscess is situated within the tonsillar parenchyma. It is rare and literature remains scarce with an incidence is 7%. Its presentation and appearance may be similar to peritonsillitis, thus making it difficult to be diagnosed and easily missed. For these reasons, the authors have chosen to discuss peritonsillitis and intratonsillar abscess, its presentation, diagnosis, and treatment.

2. Pathogenesis

2.1 Peritonsillitis

Earlier understanding is that peritonsillitis occurs secondary to acute exudative tonsillitis. After all one may argue that it is the inflammation of the tonsils due to infection which is not resolving that may develop into a surrounding soft tissue infection or abscess collections [3]. The pathogenesis of tonsillitis will not be discussed in detail within this chapter. Acute exudative tonsillitis is commonly caused by group A beta hemolytic streptococcus which appears to be seasonal in certain countries [3]. However, literature has shown that the incidence of peritonsillitis does not coincide with that of an acute upper respiratory infection and acute tonsillitis. Kordeluk at al 2011 showed that the incidence of peritonsillitis was consistent all year round compared to acute tonsillitis and upper respiratory tract infections that were seasonal, which was commoner in the first two months of the year [4]. However, the study also found a significant relationship between acute tonsillitis and peritonsillitis occurring within the same week, indicating that peritonsillitis may be caused by the same pathogen as acute tonsillitis rather than being a sequela of it.

The presence of minor salivary glands termed Weber's gland may be the culprit for infection resulting in peritonsillitis. These glands are concentrated at the upper region of the peritonsillar space at the soft palate superiorly and some may be found at the middle and inferior sections. These glands have ducts that open onto the surface of the tonsils inferiorly. Production of secretions is thought to aid cleaning of the tonsillar surface from food debris and digesting trapped food within the crypts. Tonsillitis or its inflammation causes obstructions of these ducts leading to abscess formation within the gland. These abscesses form the peritonsillar abscess superior to the tonsils at the soft palate [4, 5]. This may explain why patients post tonsillectomy do not develop peritonsillar abscess. There are two possible explanations to this, either the glands are taken out together with the tonsils during dissection or tonsillectomy has freed the obstruction from the ducts draining the Weber's glands [4–6].

2.2 Intratonsillar abscess

Unlike peritonsillitis, the occurrence of intratonsillar abscess is believed to be a sequela of acute tonsillitis. There are two postulations to the occurrence of an intratonsillar abscess. Firstly, obstruction of the tonsillar crypts and secondly delay in lymphatic flow within the tonsils. In the earlier, tonsillar inflammation may cause direct extension to the crypts, causing it to be inflamed and obstructed. Presence of debris and localized infection results in multiple abscesses with the crypts. Furthermore, failure of contraction of the tonsillopharyngeous muscle prevents expulsion of debris within these crypts.

In the second cause, the tonsils are rich in blood supply and lymphatics. They may carry bacteria to the tonsils via hematologic or lymphatic route, resulting in a localized infection. Inflammation causes reduction in lymphatic flow, leading to stasis allowing the formation of a nidus of infection within the tonsils. Inflammation intensifies leading to necrosis and abscess formation. Combination of multiple small locules of abscess may form a large abscess collection within the tonsils. This may extend into the parenchyma. Therefore, intratonsillar abscess may occur concurrently with peritonsilitis [7].

Histopathology findings suggest that bacteria travel from the surface to the crypts and underlying parenchyma via valveless lymphatic flow. Lymphatic valves are thought to be present within the capsule and absent within the parenchyma. In healthy tonsils, lymphatic clearance occurs between 10 to 30 minutes, often too short for bacteria to proliferate. However, inflammation reduces these transit times allowing a medium and environment for bacterial proliferation [7, 8].

It is important to note that with the lack of imaging years ago, earlier intratonsillar abscesses were found incidentally from histopathological examination of the tonsils post tonsillectomy among patients with peritonsillitis undergoing a hot tonsillectomy [9]. Histology revealed abscesses within crypts extending to the parenchyma, presence of necrosis within the tonsils and microabscesses [9]. **Table 1** below describes the differences in histology among tonsillitis, peritonsillitis and intratonsillar abscess [7].

Tonsillitis	Peritonsillitis	Intratonsillar abscess
Ulceration on squamous surface epithelium with neutrophils invasion	Ulceration on squamous surface epithelium with localized infiltration by neutrophils. Normal tonsillar parenchyma. Presence of neutrophils at peritonsillar space	ulceration of squamous surface epithelium. Localized infiltration of neutrophils extending into crypts. Abscess within parenchyma.

Table 1.
Differences in histology between tonsillitis, peritonsillitis and intratonsillar abscess.

2.3 Other causes

Dehydration has a role to play in peritonsillitis and intratonsillar abscess. One must not overlook other adjacent sources which are dental hygiene and sinus infections. Dental caries may be the source of infection more so in children. The authors have seen many children with recurrent tonsillitis, only to have their frequency improved by identifying and managing their oral hygiene. Furthermore, poorly controlled sinus related infections may be a culprit. Patients with allergic rhinitis may be predisposed to chronic rhinosinusitis and recurrent upper respiratory tract infection. This acts as a nidus of infection which may easily spread to the pharynx via a postnasal drip.

3. Symptomatology

Similar to tonsillitis, common symptoms of peritonsillitis and intratonsillar abscess are sore, throat, odynophagia and referred otalgia. Referred otalgia also known as secondary otalgia is a referred pain due to the glossopharyngeal nerve innervation of the tonsils and pharynx. This pain is then referred to the medial aspect of the tympanic membrane via the Jacobson's nerve [10, 11]. In tonsillitis the tonsils are erythematous and often bilateral.

In a peritonsillar abscess the soft palate is often inflamed with uvula deviation (**Figure 1**). This is often referred to as a curtain sign. This may easily be mistaken by medialization of the tonsils due to a space occupying lesion within the paraphryngeal space or deep neck abscess pushing the ipsilateral tonsils and lateral pharyngeal wall

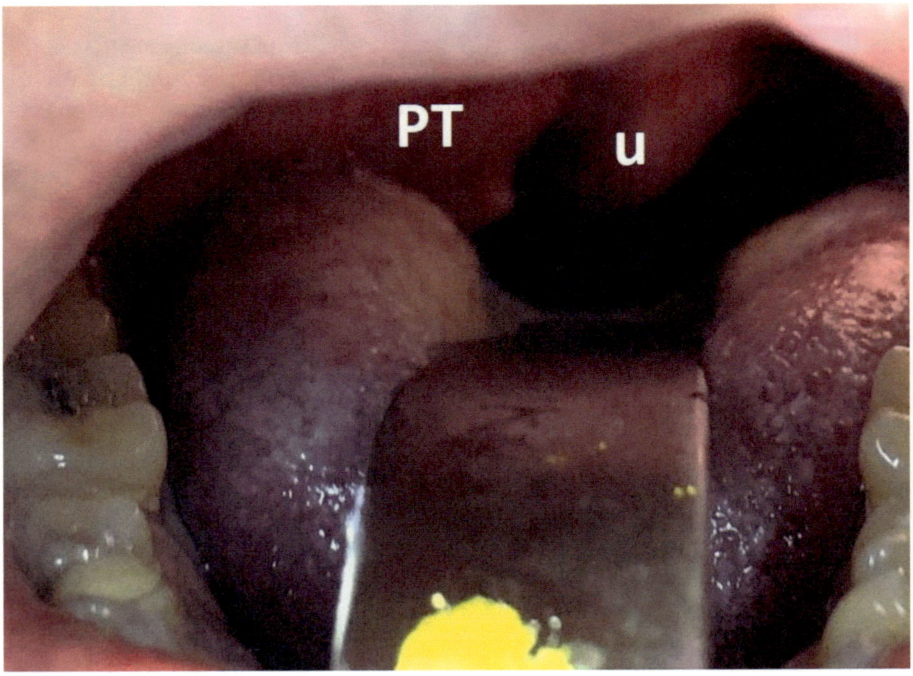

Figure 1.
Inflamed right peritonsillar region (PT) with inflamed soft palate touching the uvula (u). The tonsils were not inflamed. Image curtesy of HS Gendeh.

Fever
Trismus
Deviation of uvula
Referred pain

Table 2.
Shared symptoms of peritonsillitis and intratonsillar abscess [9].

medially. Voice change or a hot potato voice is commoner in peritonsillitis as the edematous soft palate does not assist with phonation [6, 9]. Fever is common due to systemic infection [9]. Trismus may occur too especially when there is spread of abscess of cellulitis involving the pterygoids.

In intratonsillar abscess the tonsils may be inflamed with a unilateral enlargement. Uvula deviation is unlikely for an intratonsillar abscess. Furthermore, the soft palate may or may not be oedematous depending on the presence of a concomitant peritonsillitis [6, 9]. Like peritonsillitis, trismus may occur too.

Therefore, many signs and symptoms are shared between peritonsillitis and intratonsillar abscess with no clear demarcation. For these reasons, a CT neck is always recommended when an intratonsillar abscess is suspected. Surprisingly, symptom progression is faster among patients with peritonsillar abscess compared to intratonsillar abscess [12]. Recent publication by Ahmed Ali et al. 2019 had attempted to shed some light in differentiating the symptomatology of peritonsillar abscess and intratonsillar abscess. They found that patients with peritonsillar abscess are more likely to complain of otalgia, trismus and voice change compared to neck pain which was commoner in the intratonsillar abscess group. The latter may experience higher rates of cervical lymphadenopathy due to longer presentation of symptoms; contributing to neck pain [12]. Trismus should be less among the intratonsillar abscess as the abscess should lie within the tonsillar parenchyma and not spreading to the masseteric space. Shall an intratonsillar abscess present with trismus this could be due to complication due to disease extension of soft tissue oedema to these surrounding vital structures (**Table 2**).

4. Management

The management of a patient with peritonsillitis or intratonsillar abscess ranges from bedside examination to a hot tonsillectomy. It is vital to differentiate the two due to their different management.

4.1 Clinical examination

Clinical examination is vital. A good oral examination with a headlight or adequate light source will allow the doctor to evaluate if there is any tonsillar swelling. Kindly lookout for a unilateral or bilateral swelling (**Figure 2**). Bilateral tonsils may be inflamed, enlarged with or without exudates in cases of tonsillitis. The oral cavity is examined for soft palate inflammation and/or uvula deviation. Dentition is assessed for caries which may be a source of infection especially for children. Some patients may have halitosis due to salivary stasis from reduced swallowing. If there are rhinitis symptoms, a nasal endoscopy will be useful to rule or rhinosinusitis. Examination of the neck may reveal lymphadenitis. Large swelling may suggest a deep space collection.

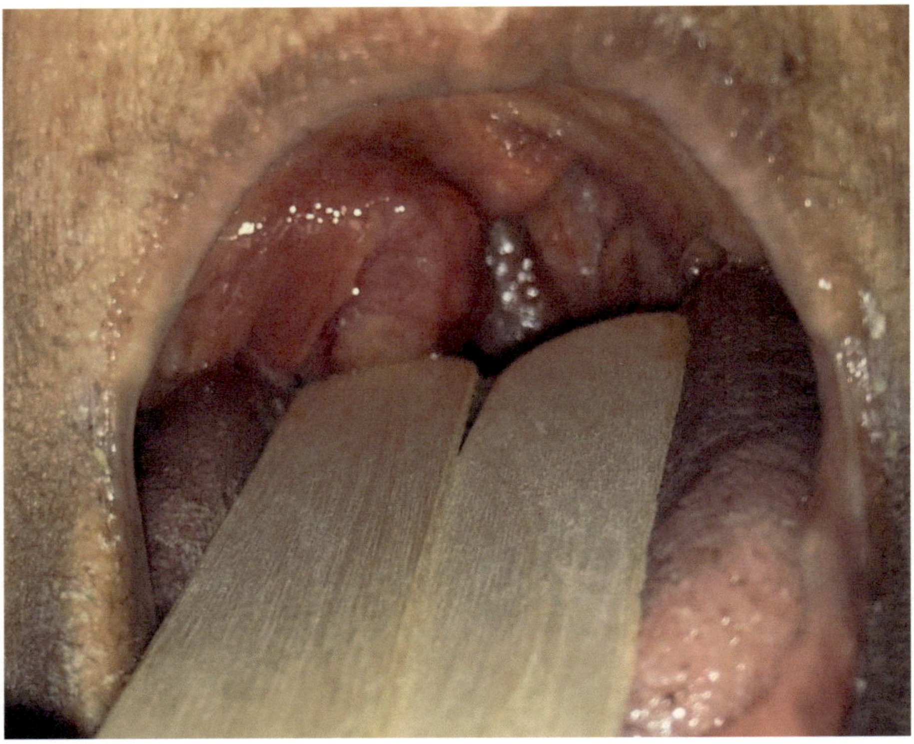

Figure 2.
An elderly lady presented with odynophagia for 3 months. Examination revealed an enlarged right tonsil with smooth surface. She had no history or indications of an infective process and malignancy should be suspected. Right tonsillar biopsy revealed a right tonsillar malignancy. Picture curtesy of HS Gendeh.

4.2 Bedside needle aspiration

When there is swelling and erythema of the soft palate and a peritonsillar abscess is suspected, a needle aspiration can be attempted as both diagnostic and therapeutic. Drainage is the gold standard for peritonsillar abscess. The area of aspiration should be that of the most fluctuant below the horizontal imaginary line of the soft palate and medial to the vertical imaginary line of the anterior pillar. The needle should be inserted straight and not laterally whereby the carotid artery is located (**Figure 3**). Depth should not be beyond 0.8 cm [13]. In order to prevent further insertion, the proximal two thirds of the needle may be lined with tape, or some have suggested the use of a needle guard whereby its distal third has been trimmed [13]. If the initial aspiration has failed, this can be tried again at lower levels above the tonsils. If successful, pus will be aspirated into the syringe, which can be sent for culture and sensitivity.

A needle aspiration is also useful when a diagnosis is uncertain. Aspiration of pus is both diagnostics confirming a peritonsillar abscess from a peritonsillar cellulitis and therapeutic. A needle aspiration is also useful when a Computed Tomography (CT) scan is hard to come by for confirmation of a peritonsillar collection. However, a needle aspiration may miss a collection with a false negative rate of 10 to 24% [14]. In such cases, if still in doubt it is wise to admit the patient and treat the patient with antibiotics or consider imaging shall the patients symptoms worsen or not respond to antibiotics. Ophir et al. suggested that all patients with peritonsillar swelling, should

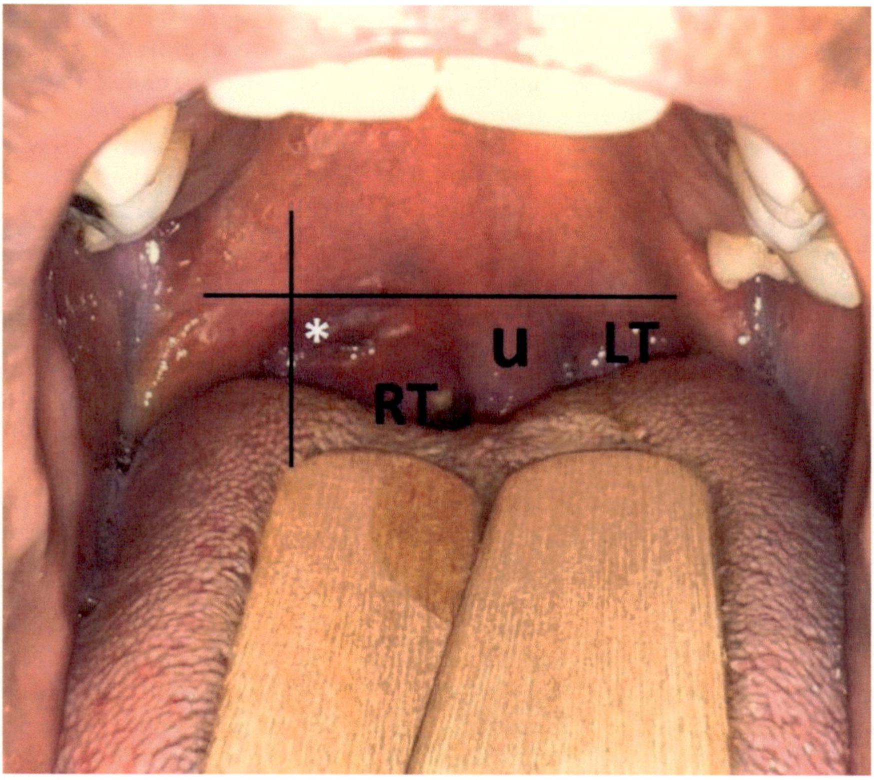

Figure 3.
*The area for needle aspiration for left tonsillar abscess should be at the area of most fluctuant below the horizontal imaginary line of the soft palate and medial to the vertical imaginary line of the anterior pillar labeled *. U: Uvula; RT: Right tonsils; LT: Left tonsils. Picture curtesy of HS Gendeh.*

undergo a needle aspiration. Shall there be no yield on three sides, thus a diagnosis of peritonsillar cellulitis is made [15].

Many have advocated needle aspiration for an intratonsillar abscess with or without imaging guidance. Without imaging guidance, the needle shall be placed at the medial border of the tonsils and directed laterally without crossing the lateral border of the tonsils. Approximately 63% of patients with intratonsillar abscess received needle aspiration with a 15% success rate [12].

4.3 Incision and drainage

For an incision and drainage, the patient should be seated to prevent aspiration of pus. A suction is handy to aspirate the pus. A 11-size blade is prepared. The authors prefer securing the proximal end of the blade with tape exposing the distal 5 mm of the blade [16]. This is to ensure that the blade does not penetrate too deep beyond the abscess. Local anesthesia may be injected or applied topically with a spray. Similarly, a small incision is made at the most fluctuant are below the horizontal imaginary line of the soft palate and medial to the vertical imaginary line of the anterior pillar. Alternatively, if a needle aspiration was successful prior, the incision should be made at the site of aspiration. A sinus forceps can be used to widen and break the loci. The patient is then required to gargle his or her oral cavity. Bear in mind that the incision site may close and will be required to be reopened from time to time to allow complete drainage and prevent re-accumulation of pus. Some have suggested flushing the cavity with a bactericidal solution using a syringe and cannula void of its inner needle. However, the authors do not recommend it nor is it recommended to insert a ribbon gauze to keep the cavity open.

What happens if both needle aspiration and incision and drainage fail to yield any pus collection? There are three possibilities being site of aspiration and incision did not target the loci of collection, the patient has peritonsillitis rather than a peritonsillar abscess, the patient may be suffering from an intratonsillar abscess. At this conjecture, one may consider giving some time for intravenous antibiotics to work. Should the swelling not reduce, or symptoms worsen, imaging should be considered to rule out the possibilities. The evidence of when to perform imaging is still lacking and it is not wrong to perform imaging earlier when no yield is obtained.

Incision and drainage can be performed for intratonsillar abscess not responding to treatment or failed a needle aspiration. Th incision should be made at the medial surface of the tonsils directed towards its center avoiding its lateral border.

Contraindications to a needle aspiration and incision and drainage are a severe trismus. The above two can be done under local anesthesia for an adult. However, for children, it is certainly recommended to be performed under general anesthesia.

4.4 Imaging

In the earlier years, imaging used to be reserved for peritonsillitis not responding to treatment or if there are suspicions of complication a deep neck abscess. However, the improved and easier access to CT imaging in tertiary referral centers have resulted in imaging to be performed even before treatment is initiated with antimicrobial therapy or needle aspiration. Clinical diagnosis of peritonsillitis has a sensitivity of 78% and specificity of 50% when compared to CT imaging [17]. The authors would reserve imaging where a peritonsillitis is not resolving or worsening with antibiotics despite negative aspiration. In other words, when a peritonsillar cellulitis diagnosis is in doubt. Contrast CT of the head and neck may indicate a rim enhancing collection superior to the tonsil in a peritonsillar abscess or within the tonsils in an intratonsillar abscess (**Figure 4**). There may be surrounding soft tissue oedema and cervical lymphadenopathy. On the other hand, intra tonsillar abscess diagnosis often requires imaging for confirmation [12]. This may explain the underdiagnosing and under reporting of intratonsillar abscess prior to this due to the more cautious use of imaging.

Neck radiographs have little value in diagnosing peritonsillitis or intratonsillar abscess. It may be useful to identify a retropharyngeal abscess as a complication. Shall there be a retropharyngeal abscess, a CT is often required to identify extension, spread and drainage approach [18, 19].

Ultrasonography on the other hand has proven to be effective in differentiating a peritonsillar cellulitis and abscess in the emergency department upon presentation [17]. Presence of fluid within the posterior pharynx can be identified/It is also handy to guide a needle aspiration of a peritonsillar abscess which is both diagnostic and therapeutic, more so for smaller loci. Some have even reported the use of ultrasonography in the emergency department to drain the abscess and discharge the patient with antibiotics without further complications [14]. The downside of ultrasonography is it is operator dependent and ENT surgeons may not be trained in using them.

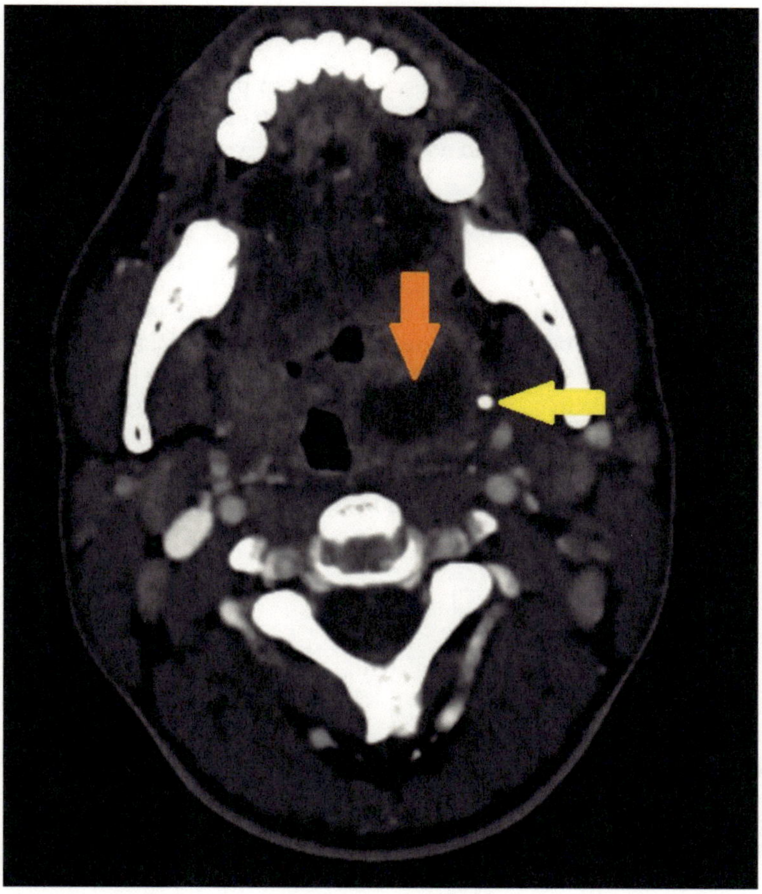

Figure 4.
Contrasted axial CT neck showing a rim enhancing hypodence collection of the left palatine tonsil (orange arrow) representing a left intratonsillar abscess. Note the lateral calcification (yellow arrow) representing a tonsilolith. A tonsilolith may cause obstruction to the lymphatic outflow of the tonsils resulting in an intratonsillar abscess. Image curtesy of HS Gendeh.

4.5 Intravenous antibiotics

Among 48 aspirations of peritonsillar abscess, there were 58 anaerobic and 49 aerobic bacteria isolated. Among the aerobic group, streptococcus group, Haemophilus group and staph aureus are the organisms isolated. Anaerobes are common owing to their presence in the oral cavity. Many patients had a combination of aerobes and anaerobes. Moreover, more than half of the specimens had B lactamase producing organisms resistant to penicillin [20]. Klung et al. revealed that the most common bacteria were streptococcus viridans, Group A beta haemolytic streptococcus, F necrophorum and staph aureus [21]. Co-amoxiclav is the most prescribed antibiotic followed by clindamycin. Duration of antibiotics ranged from five to fourteen days with 10 days being most popular [22]. Many authors have recommended a broad-spectrum antibiotic with or without metronidazole or penicillin with a second antibiotic with b lactamase activity. Certainly, due to its rarity there has yet to be recommendations for intratonsillar abscess [20].

5. Intravenous fluids

Patients presenting with a peritonsillar cellulitis or peritonsillar abscess may be septic. They may have odynophagia with a decrease in oral intake. Therefore, hydration assessment is important and do not hesitate to convene intravenous fluids as appropriately.

5.1 Tonsillectomy

A tonsillectomy performed during an ongoing infection of a peritonsillitis or intratonsillar abscess is term an immediate or hot tonsillectomy. Earlier literature recommended a hot tonsillectomy as a treatment of the above two [23]. However, recent evidence suggests that adequate drainage of collection of a peritonsillitis or intratonsillar abscess with systemic antibiotics is sufficient to resolve infection. Therefore, the authors have never required to perform a hot tonsillectomy for the above two indications in their institution. Only once a hot tonsillectomy had to be performed for a non-resolving

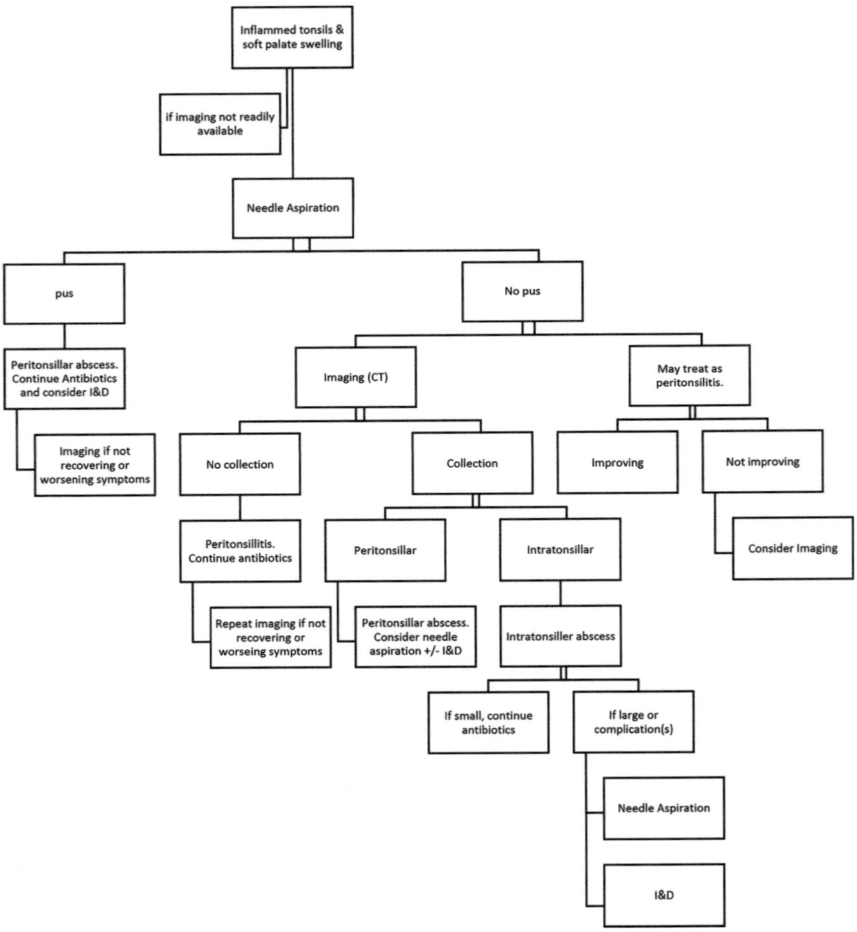

Figure 5.
A suggested flow chart on the management in identifying a peritonsillar abscess and an intratonsillar abscess. I&D; incision and drainage.

tonsillitis with pyrexia despite being on prolonged intravenous antibiotics. The risk of a hot tonsillectomy is bleeding due to ongoing inflammation and infection. Certainly, the availability of powered instruments such as an ultrasonic scalpel does reduce this risk.

An elective tonsillectomy should be considered among patients with recurrent peritonsillar abscess or recurrent peritonsillar abscess twice or more. Some authors have suggested that a single episode is sufficient to warrant an elective tonsillectomy. This is because 90% of patients with peritonsillar abscess do not have recurrence [24]. In summary, **Figure 5** depicts a flow chart on the management in identifying a peritonsillar abscess and an intratonsillar abscess.

6. Complications

6.1 Upper airway obstruction

A large collection has a potential to cause upper airway obstruction, more so if it is complicated with a retropharyngeal abscess. This is an emergency, and the airway must be secured first.

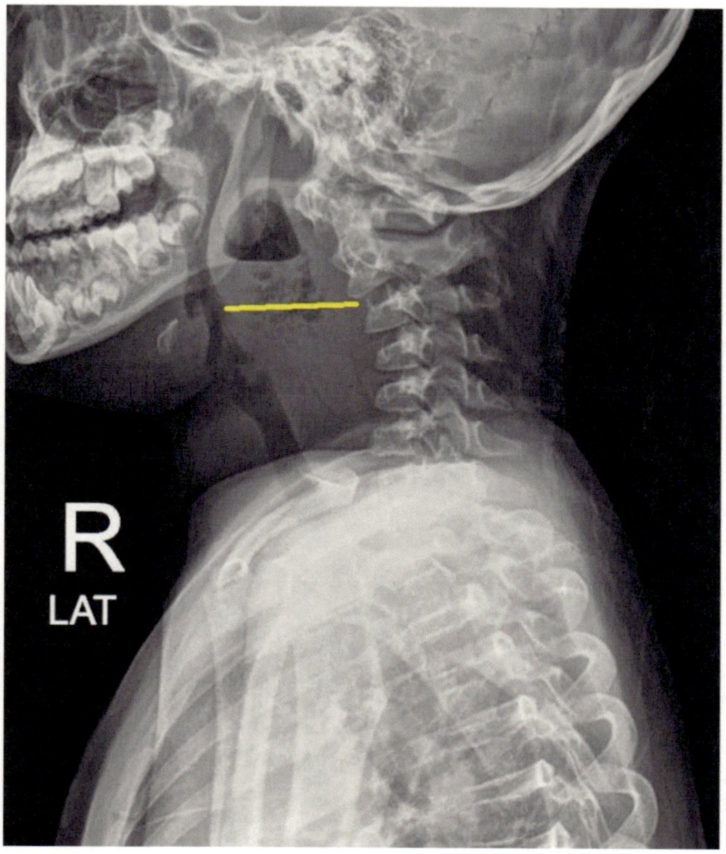

Figure 6.
Lateral neck radiograph of a child with retropharyngeal abscess. Appreciate the increase in horizontal distance between the pharynx anteriorly and vertebrae posteriorly. The posterior pharyngeal wall is pushed anteriorly. Picture curtesy of HS Gendeh.

6.2 Retropharyngeal abscess, parapharyngeal abscess, mediastinitis

A retropharyngeal lymph node drains lymphatics from the posterior part of the nose, nasopharynx, and adenoids. Therefore, infection from the palatine tonsils may spread retrogradely to the retropharyngeal lymph nodes. Suppuration of these lymph nodes results in a retropharyngeal abscess [25]. The left and right retropharyngeal spaces are in communication; thus, the patient may have a bulge in the posterior pharyngeal wall (**Figure 6**). Airway compromise may occur if severe enough.

The retropharyngeal space spreads from the skull base cranially to the posterior mediastinum caudally. Therefore, if severe enough it may be a pathway to mediastinitis [25]. Buccopharyngeal fascia forms the anterior boundary while the prevertebral fascia forms the posterior boundary.

The retropharyngeal space connects directly to the parapharyngeal space. The Parapharyngeal space is a potential space containing lymph nodes that may undergo suppuration. It is not surprised that peritonsillar retropharyngeal and parapharyngeal infections are termed deep neck infections.

6.3 Intracranial involvement

Very rarely would a patient present with intracranial complications. However, local spread of infection may result in cavernous sinus thrombosis, brain abscess, meningitis, or osteomyelitis of the sella turcica.

6.4 Recurrent abscess

Recurrent abscess is reported to be in 15% and 7% for peritonsillar abscess and intratonsillar abscess respectively. Limited case reports of ipsilateral brain abscess and peritonsillar abscess [26].

7. Conclusion

The presence of minor salivary glands termed Weber's gland may be the culprit for infection resulting in peritonsillitis. An intratonsillar abscess occurs when the abscess is situated within the tonsillar parenchyma and may occur concurrently with peritonsilitis. Dehydration has a role to play in peritonsillitis and intratonsillar abscess and the medical therapy consists of intravenous antibiotics and intravenous fluids. Poor management can result in complications like retropharyngeal abscess, parapharyngeal abscess, mediastinitis and upper airway obstruction and CT scan with contrast is essential to know its extension, spread and drainage approaches. Aspiration of pus is diagnostic confirming a peritonsillar abscess from a peritonsillar cellulitis. Incision and drainage can be performed for intratonsillar abscess not responding to treatment or a failed needle aspiration which is preferably performed under general anesthesia for children. Elective tonsillectomy should be indicated for patients with recurrent peritonsillar abscess. Thus, a clear understanding of peritonsillitis and intratonsillar abscess, its presentation, diagnosis and treatment is of outmost importance to physicians dealing with the airway and food passageway.

Author details

Hardip Singh Gendeh[1*] and Balwant Singh Gendeh[1,2]

1 Department of Otorhinolaryngology, Head and Neck Surgery, Universiti Kebangsaan Malaysia Medical Center, Malaysia

2 Pantai Hospital Kuala Lumpur, Malaysia

*Address all correspondence to: hardip88@gmail.com

References

[1] Crumbie L, Chaves C. Waldeyer Ring. Available from: https://www.kenhub.com/en/library/anatomy/waldeyers-ring [Accessed: March 6, 2023]

[2] Fried MP, Forrest JL. Peritonsillitis: Evaluation of current therapy. Archives of Otolaryngology. 1981;**107**(5):283-286. DOI: 10.1001/archotol.1981.00790410021004

[3] Woolley BJWAL. Cummings Otolaryngology Head & Neck Surgery. St Louis, MO: Mosby; 2005

[4] Kordeluk S, Novack L, Puterman M, Kraus M, Joshua BZ. Relation between peritonsillar infection and acute tonsillitis: Myth or reality? Otolaryngology and Head and Neck Surgery. 2011;**145**(6):940-945

[5] Galioto JN. Peritonsillar Abscess. American Family Physician. 2017;**95**(8):501-506

[6] Powell EL, Powell J, Samuel JR, Wilson JA. A review of the pathogenesis of adult peritonsillar abscess: Time for a re-evaluation. The Journal of Antimicrobial Chemotherapy. 2013;**68**(9):1941-1950

[7] Blair AB, Booth R, Baugh R. A unifying theory of tonsillitis, intratonsillar abscess and peritonsillar abscess. American Journal of Otolaryngology. 2015;**36**(4):517-520

[8] Loo BW Jr, Draney MT, Sivanandan R, Ruehm SG, Pawlicki T, Xing L, et al. Indirect MR lymphangiography of the head and neck using conventional gadolinium contrast: A pilot study in humans. International Journal of Radiation Oncology, Biology, Physics. 2006;**66**(2):462-468

[9] Childs EW, Baugh RF, Diaz JA. Tonsillar abscess. Journal of the National Medical Association. 1991;**83**(4):333-336

[10] Chen RC, Khorsandi AS, Shatzkes DR, Holliday RA. The radiology of referred otalgia. AJNR. American Journal of Neuroradiology. 2009;**30**(10):1817-1823

[11] Greenhall CJ, Rhys R. The radiology of referred otalgia. American Journal of Neuroradiology. 2014;**23**(2):1817-1823

[12] Ali SA, Kovatch KJ, Smith J, Bellile EL, Hanks JE, Truesdale CM, et al. Predictors of intratonsillar versus peritonsillar abscess: A case-control series. The Laryngoscope. 2019;**129**(6):1354-1359

[13] Roberts JRMD. InFocus: Mastering aspiration for Peritonsillar abscess. Emergency Medicine News. 2018;**40**(12):8-9

[14] Lyon M, Blaivas M. Intraoral ultrasound in the diagnosis and treatment of suspected peritonsillar abscess in the emergency department. Academic Emergency Medicine. 2005;**12**:85Y88

[15] Ophir D, Bawnik J, Poria Y, Porat M, Marshak G. Peritonsillar abscess. A prospective evaluation of outpatient management by needle aspiration. Archives of Otolaryngology, Head and Neck Surgery. 1988;**114**:661-663

[16] Gupta G, McDowell RH. Peritonsillar Abscess. Treasure Island (FL): StatPearls Publishing; 2022

[17] Scott PM, Loftus WK, Kew J, et al. Diagnosis of peritonsillar infections: A prospective study of ultrasound, computerized tomography and clinical

diagnosis. The Journal of Laryngology and Otology. 1999;**113**:229Y232

[18] Honnegowda T, Silvia WD, Babu VS. Clinical evaluation and management of deep neck space infections. International Journal of Head and Neck Surgery. 2017;**8**(3):102-106

[19] Sakaguchi M, Sato S, Asawa S, Taguchi K. Computed tomographic findings in peritonsillar abscess and cellulitis. The Journal of Laryngology & Otology. 1995;**109**(5):449-451

[20] Brook I, Frazier EH, Thompson DH. Aerobic and anaerobic microbiology of peritonsillar abscess. The Laryngoscope. 1991;**101**(3):289-292

[21] Klug TE, Greve T, Hentze M. Complications of peritonsillar abscess. Annals of Clinical Microbiology and Antimicrobials. 2020;**19**(1):32

[22] Wu V, Manojlovic Kolarski M, Kandel CE, Monteiro E, Chan Y. Current trend of antibiotic prescription and management for peritonsillar abscess: A cross-sectional study. Laryngoscope Investigative Otolaryngology. 2021;**6**(2):183-187

[23] Hsu C-H, Lin Y-S, Lee J-C. Intratonsillar abscess. Otolaryngology-Head and Neck Surgery. 2008;**139**(6):861-862

[24] Powell J, Wilson JA. An evidence-based review of peritonsillar abscess. Clinical Otolaryngology. 2012;**37**:136-145. DOI: 10.1111/j.1749-4486.2012.02452.x

[25] Esposito S, De Guido C, Pappalardo M, Laudisio S, Meccariello G, Capoferri G, et al. Retropharyngeal, Parapharyngeal and Peritonsillar abscesses. Children (Basel). 2022;**9**(5):618

[26] Sankararaman S, Riel-Romero RM, Gonzalez-Toledo E. Brain abscess from a peritonsillar abscess in an immunocompetent child: A case report and review of the literature. Pediatric Neurology. 2012;**47**(6):451-454

Chapter 3

Evolution of Adenoid Surgery

Anubhuti Dhanuka, Anukaran Mahajan, Karunesh Gupta and Stuti Mahajan

Abstract

Adenoid, also known as the Luschka's or nasopharyngeal tonsil, is a mass of lymphoid tissue located in the roof of nasopharynx. The term 'adenoid' was coined by Meyer. Earliest records of adenoid surgery date back to 1842, when Yearsley reported removal of mucus membrane from behind the uvula to improve ear function. Other techniques for adenoidectomy included bare fingernails or finger ring knife, which are considered obsolete now. From mid-1930s to early 1960s, radiation therapy of the adenoid was used extensively. Transoral adenoid curetting and electrical dissection techniques followed and became mainstay of treatment for a long time. Infact, these are still in use in many centres across the world. Like any other surgery, introduction of nasal endoscopes and powered instruments revolutionised adenoid surgery by greatly increasing the precision and minimising collateral damage. Plasma-mediated ablation (Coblation) promises 'blood-less' surgery. Presently, the trend is focussed towards using powered instruments (Microdebrider and/or Coblation) under endoscopic visualisation for complete adenoidectomy.

Keywords: adenoid, adenoidectomy, coblation, microdebrider, adenoid curette

1. Introduction

The adenoid forms part of Waldeyer's ring of lymphoid tissue at the portal of the upper respiratory tract. In early childhood this is the first site of immunological contact for inhaled antigens. Santorini was the first one to describe the nasopharyngeal lymphoid aggregate or 'Luschka's tonsil' in 1724. Wilhelm Meyer coined the term 'adenoid' to apply to 'nasopharyngeal vegetations' in 1870.

Adenoid hypertrophy is considered to be a culprit of upper airway obstruction, a focus of sepsis, and persistence of otitis media with effusion.

2. Development and anatomy of the adenoid

Earliest identification of lymphoid tissue can be made at 4- to 6-weeks of gestational period, lying within the mucous membrane of nasopharynx. The adenoid is clearly identified at third month of gestation.

Adenoid tissue is anatomically located in the roof of posterior wall of nasopharynx. It can extend to the fossa of Rosenmüller and to the Eustachian tube orifice as Gerlach's tonsil. Non- keratinised stratified squamous epithelium is the lining epithelium of adenoid tissue. The arterial supply is mainly from the branches of facial artery, maxillary artery and thyrocervical trunk. Venous drainage is to the internal jugular and facial veins. Lymphatics drain into retropharyngeal lymph nodes and upper deep cervical nodes, especially the posterior triangle of the neck.

Nerve supply is from sensory branches of CN IX (Glossopharyngeal Nerve) and CN X (Vagus Nerve) [1].

Adenoid is visible using magnetic resonance imaging (MRI) from the age of 4 months in approximately 18% of the paediatric population [2]. At the age of 5 months, adenoid is identifiable in almost all children. Adenoid continues to grow rapidly during infancy and the growth plateaus between the ages of 2 and 14 years. Regression of adenoid occurs quite rapidly after 15 years of age in majority of the children. Adenoid is at the relative largest size in relation to the volume of the nasopharynx in the 7-year old age group [3]. Clinical symptoms are more common in younger age groups, due to relatively small volume of nasopharynx and the increased frequency of upper respiratory tract infections (**Figures 1** and **2**).

3. Immune function of the adenoid

The function of the lymphoid tissue of Waldeyer's ring is production of antibodies. Adenoid produces B-cells, which gives rise to IgG and IgA plasma cells. Exposure to antigens via the oral and nasal route is an important part of natural acquired immunity in early childhood. Adenoid appears to have an important role in the development of 'immunological memory' in younger children [4]. While some studies have found that adenoidectomy in early childhood can be immunologically undesirable [5].

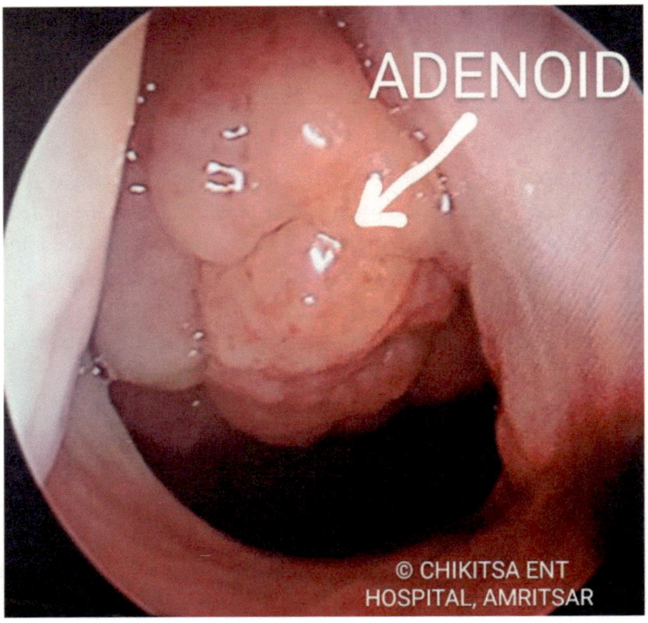

Figure 1.
Endocsopic view of adenoid tissue in nasopharynx. © Chikitsa ENT hospital, Amritsar. Used with permission.

DOI: http://dx.doi.org/10.5772/intechopen.1001462

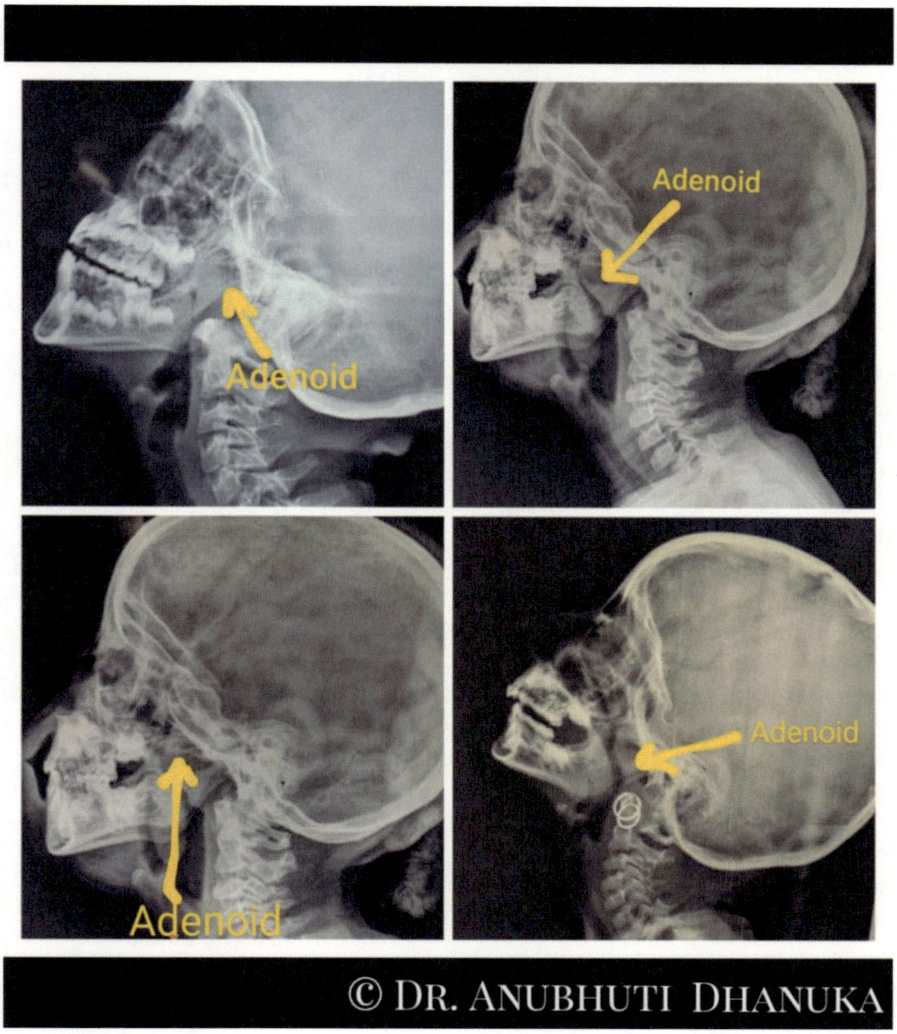

Figure 2.
X-ray nasopharynx (lateral view) showing adenoid hypertrophy.

Other studies have concluded that adenotonsillectomy does not cause significant immune deficiency [6].

Nevertheless, a careful decision has to be made for every patient individually whether to perform adenoidectomy or not.

4. Pathological effects of the adenoid

Pathological manifestations of adenoid include adenoiditis, rhinitis, rhinosinusitis, otitis media and otitis media with effusion [7].

The adenoid, due its anatomical position, is implicated in upper respiratory tract diseases due to partial or complete obstruction of the nasal choanae or as a result of sepsis. This also causes severe sleep disturbances in children. It is also a common cause of obstructive sleep apnea (OSA). Sleep- disordered breathing and habitual snoring, results in neurobehavioural morbidity, poor academic performance and hyperactive behaviour [8, 9]. The respiratory improvement following adenotonsillectomy also results in a significant increase in serum insulin-like growth factor-1 (IGF-1) [10], accounting in part for the frequently observed growth spurt following surgery.

Additionally, adenoidal hyperplasia may reduce olfactory sensitivity and, in particular, retronasal smell and taste, which improves following adenoidectomy [11].

Adenoid mass is the most common culprit for recurrent otitis media with effusion (OME) episodes in paediatric population. Owing to its proximity to the eustachian tube orifice in nasopharynx, it can cause its anatomical obstruction. Moreover, adenoid tissue acts as source of bacterial harborization and 'biofilm' formation. Recurrent acute and chronic inflammation of the adenoid and increased bacterial load (especially Haemophilus influenzae) [12–14], contributes in a more severe way to OME episodes.

As adenoid acts as a reservoir for pathogenic bacteria, it also contributes in a major way to rhinosinusitis, especially in children [15]. 'Biofilm' formation is particularly implicated in failure of medical therapy for chronic rhinosinusitis in children with adenoid hypertrophy.

Extremely rarely, Non-Hodgkin's lymphoma can also develop in the adenoid tissue [16]. Atypical lymphadenopathy, with persistent and asymmetric enlargement of the adenoid, in the absence of infection is suspicious and should prompt early imaging and biopsy to rule out malignancy.

Thus adenoid needs to be adequately managed. Over the years, various modalities for treatment of adenoid have been developed. These include observation alone, medical therapy, radiation therapy, surgical removal or a combination of these.

5. Treatment of the adenoid

5.1 Observation (wait and watch)

Adenoid size is age dependent. Adenoid mass increases in size rapidly after birth. It reaches its maximum size by 7–10 years of age. After that, it begins to regress and gradually diminishes in size throughout adulthood [3].

Although, exceptions are not unheard of. Infact, the adenoid is at its relative largest in relation to the volume of the nasopharynx in the 7-year old age group [3]. Persisting large adenoid mass in adults, filling up the entire nasopharyngeal volume, is a common finding.

In conclusion, if the adenoid mass is small in size and relatively asymptomatic, observation alone can be taken as a standalone modality, especially in children, as there is a high chance that it might regress in due course of time.

5.2 Medical therapy

Traditionally, surgery and watchful waiting were the only viable options for symptomatic adenoid disease. There is now a evidence that topical nasal steroid sprays can cause reduction in adenoid size with improvement in symptoms, although at present that role is unclear [17].

Recent studies have proven that Vitamin D3 deficiency is linked with adenoid hypertrophy [18]. Therefore adequate supplementation of Vitamin D3 needs to be done in patients being treated for adenoid hypertrophy.

5.3 Radiation therapy

Radiation therapy for ablating adenoid mass is more of historical importance only.

From the mid-1930s to the early 1960s, radiation therapy of adenoid was in extensive use, both for children and for army aviators and navy submarine crews during WWII [19].

However, radiation therapy is a thing of past owing to its immense side effect profile and development of better and more effective treatment modalities.

5.4 Surgery for adenoid

A symptomatic adenoid often warrants its surgical removal. An ideal adenoidectomy aims at complete removal of adenoid tissue, without damaging surrounding structures (eustachian tube opening, torus tubaris, soft palate, superior constrictor muscle). Over the years various techniques for adenoidectomy have been developed, and are discussed below.

5.4.1 Evolution of adenoid surgery

The adenoid surgery has evolved over the years on the basis of visualisation of the adenoid. While the earliest documented adenoid surgeries were blind procedures, the advent of endoscopes in nasal surgeries has seen a paradigm shift in how adenoidectomy is performed today.

5.4.2 Blind procedures for adenoidectomy

5.4.2.1 Adenoid curettes and adenotomes

Since the earliest descriptions of adenoidectomy, a great number of different techniques have been described and used successfully. All of these techniques are based on the principle of adequate removal of the adenoids without damage to the surrounding structures, such as the torus tubarus, the palate, the posterior pharyngeal wall, and the choana. Recent minimally invasive and endoscopic technologies have also been applied for adenoidectomy.

The first mention of adenoidectomy was done by Meyer in 1867 [20]. He used a sharp ring curette inserted blindly through oral cavity by just palpating the 'nasopharyngeal vegetations'.

Soon after, many new methods were developed for the removal of adenoids, most of which approached the adenoids transorally.

A ring knife was invented by Gottstein in 1885 [21]. Beckmann modified this ring knife in 1897 [22]. Punch forceps and adenotome were also developed for removal of adenoid mass. Sir St Clair Thomson developed the famous adenoidectomy curette, complete with its cage to ensure safety and to entangle the tissue fragments and blood during adenoidectomy. This curette is still used in the conventional curettage adenoidectomy [23].

The current standard procedure for blind adenoidectomy is curettage. Patient is placed in Rose position and an appropriate sized mouth gag is placed in the oral cavity. St Clair Thompson adenoidectomy curette is inserted in the oral cavity, bypassing the oropharynx in order to reach the nasopharynx and is engaged at the adenoid pad. The adenoid mass is removed from superior to inferior with a single pass of the curette. Care should be taken to avoid injury to the deep muscular and vertebral plane, to the torus region or to the choanal area. The resultant adenoid bed is packed with a sponge to achieve heamostasis. Saline irrigation also helps in achieving haemostasis. Completion is confirmed by digital palpation.

The limitations of this technique is less precise removal and thus less effective treatment, increased bleeding, velopharyngeal insufficiency, and lack of surgical visualisation. Blind curettage procedure does not always completely remove the adenoid tissue, thus recurrence is common with this technique (**Figure 3**) [24].

5.4.3 Indirect visualisation using mirrors

Blind techniques of adenoidectomy were particularly accompanied by high complication rates. Damage to surrounding structures like eustachian tube caused stenosis, leading to ear problems. Soft palate injury resulted in velopharyngeal insufficiency. Superior constrictor/prevertebral injury was often accompanied by primary or secondary haemorrhages and neck stiffness. Moreover, complete adenoidectomy was seldom possible with these techniques and residual adenoid tissue was often left at upper nasopharynx, Fossa of Rosenmuller and choana [25–29].

To rectify these shortcomings, a lot of surgeons started to prefer indirect visualisation of nasopharynx using a laryngeal mirror/dental mirror introduced through oral cavity.

5.4.3.1 Microdebrider- adenoidectomy under indirect visualisation

A few surgeons started to use a curved shaver or microdebrider for adenoidectomy under continuous indirect visualisation through a laryngeal mirror [28, 30, 31]. Both the shaver and the mirror were introduced transorally. The oscillating shaver tip is under continuous visualisation while it removes adenoid tissue in a superior to inferior manner. The enhanced precision enables safe tissue removal from earlier 'inaccessible areas' like choana, upper nasopharynx and peri-tubal area.

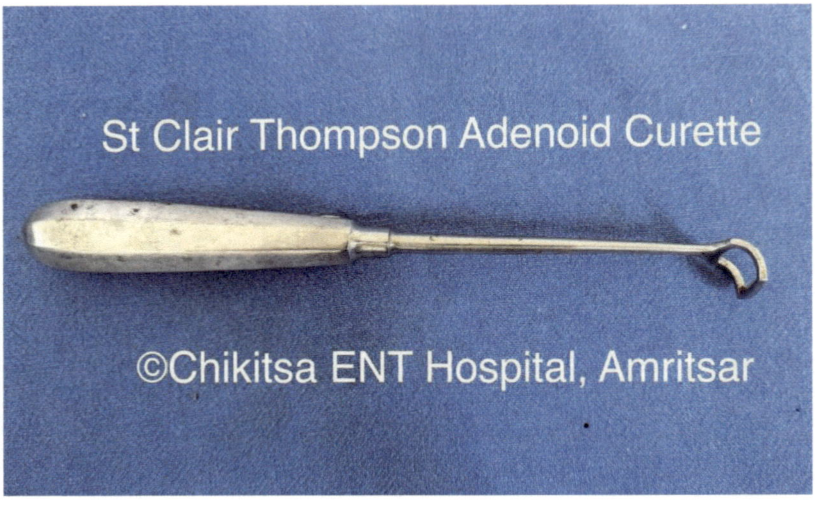

Figure 3.
St. Clair Thompson adenoidectomy curette. © Chikitsa ENT hospital, Amritsar. Used with permission.

DOI: http://dx.doi.org/10.5772/intechopen.1001462

5.4.3.2 Suction diathermy assisted adenoidectomy under indirect visualisation

A laryngeal mirror is introduced transorally to visualise adenoid mass in nasopharynx [26, 32]. Adenoid mass is ablated using an insulated, curved Frazier-type suction system or, a disposable, malleable, hand-switching suction coagulator. As the diathermy cauterises the adenoid mass, it shrinks, while the suction evacuates the smoke. This method gained widespread acceptance owing to its advantages of being precise, easy to perform, fast, bloodless and relatively inexpensive (**Figure 4**).

5.4.3.3 Laser adenoidectomy

Laser adenoidectomy, using a CO2 laser, has also been described in literature. Jaw and palate are retracted using laser-compatible retractors and lips and teeth are covered with foil. Wet towels are used to cover the rest of the face. A microscope mounted CO2 laser is then reflected onto the adenoid mass through a polished mirror kept in oropharynx. The mirror also assists in indirect visualisation of adenoid mass being ablated.

Although an interesting technique, laser adenoidectomy never gained popularity, probably owing to its greater cost, and development of better tools and techniques (Microdebrider/Coblation) [33].

5.4.4 Endoscopic visualisation

(See **Figure 5**)

5.4.4.1 Nasal endoscopic adenoid curettage

The nasal cavities and nasopharynx are examined using a 0° nasal endoscope [34]. Boyle- Davis mouth gag is used to open the mouth wide. An adenoidectomy curette is

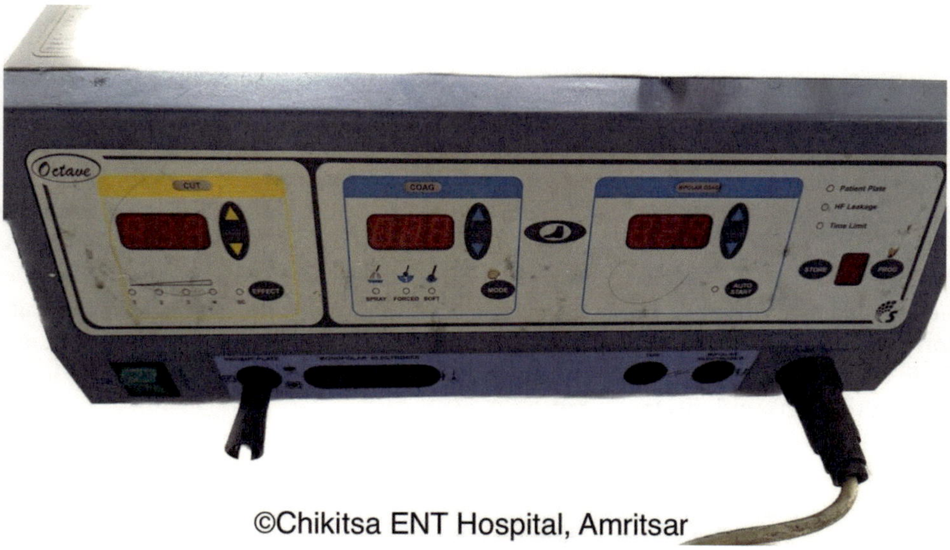

Figure 4.
Bipolar and monopolar cautery unit (diathermy). © Chikitsa ENT hospital, Amritsar. Used with permission.

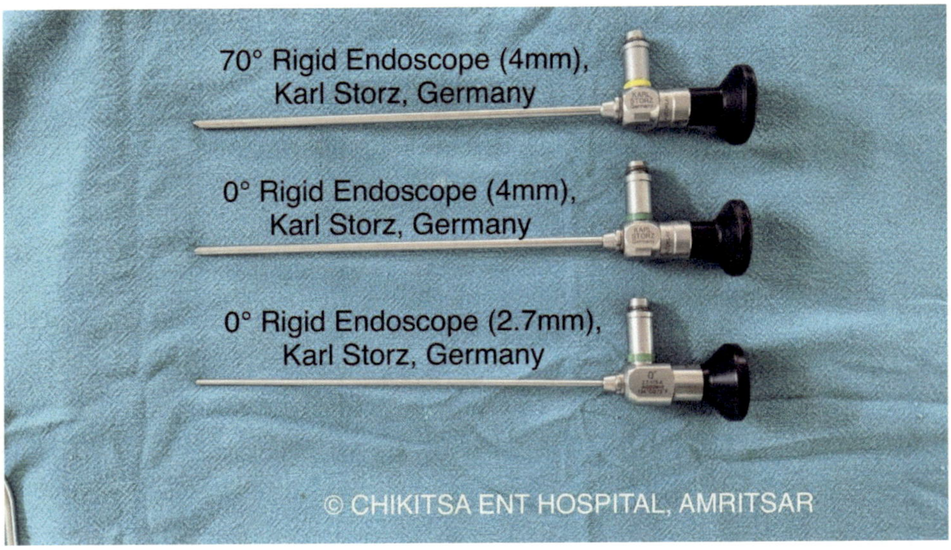

Figure 5.
Karl Storz rigid endoscopes. © Chikitsa ENT hospital, Amritsar. Used with permission.

placed into the nasopharynx via the transoral route. Under endoscopic guidance, the blade of the adenoid curette is placed just above the superior border of the adenoid. Care should be taken to avoid touching the eustachian tube on both sides. The nasal endoscope is then taken out from the nose and the curettage is done as per conventional protocol.

5.4.4.2 Transoral endoscopic adenoidectomy using suction diathermy

A 45° rigid scope is introduced into the oral cavity to the oropharynx with the camera pointing upwards to the nasopharynx [35]. A suction coagulator is introduced alongside the endoscope. Adenoidectomy is performed under direct endoscopic vision by using a combination of monopolar coagulation and suction.

5.4.4.3 Transnasal endoscopy along with powered transnasal adenoidectomy

A zero degree rigid endoscope (2.7 mm/4.0 mm) is passed through the nasal cavity to visualise adenoid mass in nasopharyhnx [27, 36]. A straight (zero degree) microdebrider blade is passed through the nasal cavity under endoscopic visualisation to reach the nasopharynx. The oscillating microdebrider blade is then switched on to debride the adenoid tissue in an anterior to posterior fashion. Continuous irrigation and suction in the microdebrider system provides for better visualisation. Its major advantage lies in clearing the adenoid tissue from around choana and eustachian tube, without injuring the surrounding structures.

5.4.4.4 Transoral endoscopy with transoral powered adenoidectomy

This approach uses a 70-degree rigid endoscope (4.0 mm) and a posterior facing- 40 degree curved microdebrider blade, both introduced through oral cavity [37].

Palate can be retracted using feeding tubes introduced through nose. The adenoid tissue is debrided and sucked by the microdebrider system. Continuous irrigation and suction of the system facilitates the process. A gauze piece is kept in the end to achieve haemostasis. This technique is considered to have a better clearance of the peritubal adenoid mass without any injury of nasal septum/turbinates.

5.4.4.5 *Transnasal endoscopy with transoral powered adenoidectomy*

Transnasal endoscopy with transoral powered (Microdebrider/Coblation) adenoidectomy is the authors' preferred technique. This technique was first described by Dr. Satish Jain (Jaipur, India) and has become now the most commonly used technique across Indian subcontinent. The patient lies in a supine position under general anaesthesia using an orotracheal tube. The head end is elevated at 15–30 degrees. A zero degree rigid endoscope (2.7 mm/4.0 mm) is used to visualise the adenoid mass in the nasopharynx. A mouth gag opens the mouth to allow introduction of powered instruments. An anterior facing −40 or 60 degree curved microdebrider blade, introduced transorally, allows for precise removal of adenoid mass under continuous endoscopic visualisation. The removal of adenoids is done in three phases. First phase allows gross debulking of the adenoid tissue. The second phase allows fine removal of adenoid tissue anterior to perimysial layer of superior constrictor muscle. While the third phase allows removal of adenoid tissue from the peritubal region (especially fossa of rosenmuller on either side) and upper nasopharynx. Coblation is then used to achieve complete haemostasis. Alternately, all three phases can be done using Coblation alone using its adenoidectomy wand. This technique has major advantages as against all other techniques in the form of better visualisation, complete removal of adenoid tissue and minimum blood loss. Eustachian tube, torus tuboris and posterior pharyngeal wall also remain well protected with this technique (**Figures 6–10**).

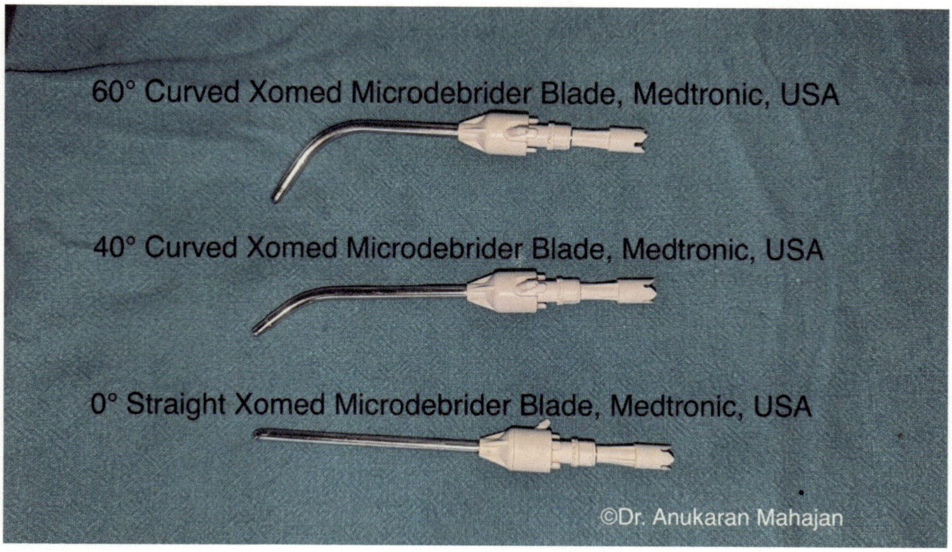

Figure 6.
Xomed microdebrider blades, curved and straight.

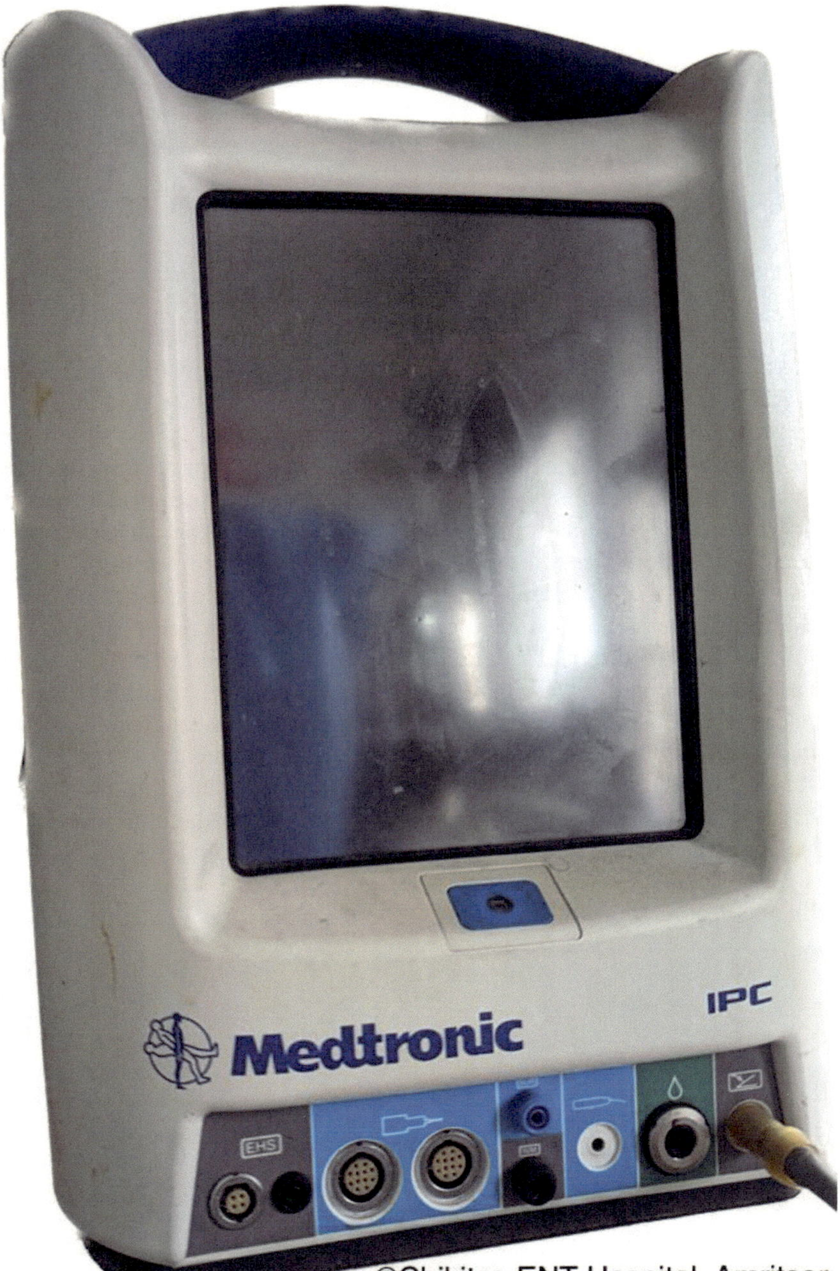

Figure 7.
IPC medtronic (USA) microdebrider unit. © Chikitsa ENT hospital, Amritsar. Used with permission.

DOI: http://dx.doi.org/10.5772/intechopen.1001462

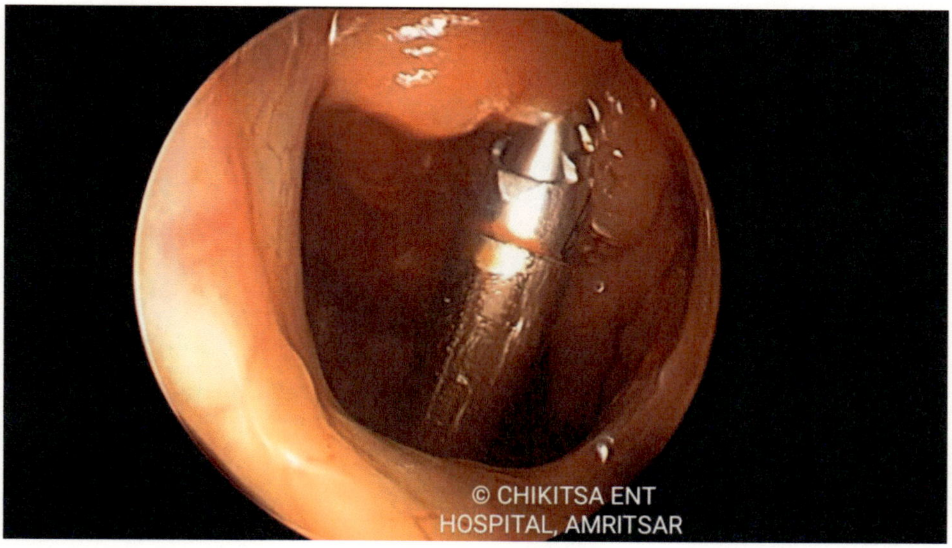

Figure 8.
Transnasal endoscopic view of transoral powered adenoidectomy using microdebrider (60° curved xomed blade). © Chikitsa ENT hospital, Amritsar. Used with permission.

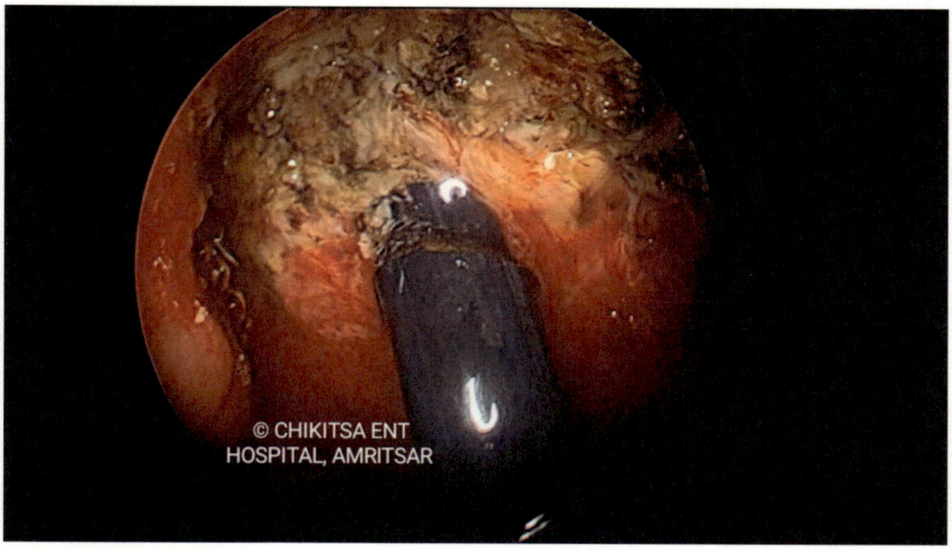

Figure 9.
Transnasal endoscopic view of transoral powered adenoidectomy using coblator. © Chikitsa ENT hospital, Amritsar. Used with permission.

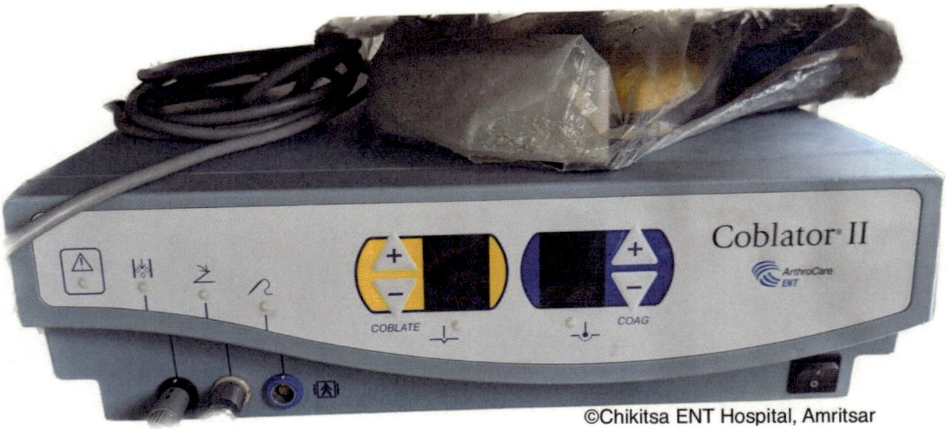

Figure 10.
Arthrocare coblator unit, Smith and Nephew (USA). © Chikitsa ENT hospital, Amritsar. Used with permission.

6. Conclusion

Adenoid is nasopharyngeal lymphatic tissue, present in all children. Symptomatic adenoid warrants treatment, more often than not, in the form of surgery. Over the decades surgical techniques and tools have evolved to make adenoidectomy a safe and effective procedure. Transnasal endoscopic visualisation with transoral powered adenoidectomy using microdebrider/coblation is the most advanced and authors' preferred method.

Acknowledgements

I wish to express my sincere gratitude towards Dr. Arun Dhanuka, Vibha Dhanuka and Dr. Aishwarya Dhanuka for their constant moral support. I am fortunate to have worked with Dr. Stuti Mahajan and Dr. Anukaran Mahajan on numerous adenoid cases. A special vote of thanks to Dr. Anupama Mahajan, HOD Anatomy and Director Principal, SGRDIMSR, Amritsar for providing valuable insight into the anatomy and pathology of this disease. I shall always be indebted to Dr. Karunesh Gupta and Dr. Rajeev Kapila for their unparalleled mentorship.

Conflict of interest

The authors declare no conflict of interest.

Author details

Anubhuti Dhanuka*, Anukaran Mahajan, Karunesh Gupta and Stuti Mahajan
Chikitsa ENT Hospital, Amritsar, India

*Address all correspondence to: anubhutidhanuka@gmail.com

References

[1] University of Texas Medical Section Grand Rounds. Tonsillitis, Tonsillectomy, and Adenoidectomy. 1999. Available from: https://www.utmb.edu/

[2] Jaw TS, Sheu RS, Liu GC, Lin WC. Development of adenoids: A study by measurement with MRI images. The Kaohsiung Journal of Medical Sciences. 1999;**15**:12-18

[3] Vogler RC, Ii FJ, Pilgram TK. Age-specific size of the normal adenoid pad on magnetic resonance imaging. Clin Otol Allied Sci. 2000;**25**:392-395

[4] Wysocka J, Hassmann E, Lipska A, Musiatowicz M. Naïve and memory T-cells in hypertrophied adenoids in children according to age. International Journal of Pediatric Otorhinolaryngology. 2003;**67**:237-241

[5] Brandtzaeg P. Immunology of the tonsils and adenoids: Everything the ENT surgeon needs to know. International Journal of Pediatric Otorhinolaryngology. 2003;**67**:69-76

[6] Ikinciogullari A, Dogu F, Ikinciogullari A, et al. Is the immune system influenced by adenotonsillectomy in children? International Journal of Pediatric Otorhinolaryngology. 2002;**66**:251-257

[7] Richardson MA. Sore throat, tonsillitis and adenoiditis. The Medical Clinics of North America. 1999;**83**:75-83

[8] Brockmann PE, Bertrand P, Pardo T, et al. Prevalence of habitual snoring and associated neurocognitive consequences among Chilean school aged children. International Journal of Pediatric Otorhinolaryngology. 2012;**76**:1327-1331

[9] Owens JA. Neurocognitive and behavioral impact of sleep disordered breathing in children. Pediatrics Pulm. 2009;**44**:417-422

[10] Bar A, Tarasuik A, Segev Y, et al. The effect of adenotonsillectomy on serum insulin like growth factor-I and growth in children with obstructive sleep apnea syndrome. The Journal of Pediatrics. 1999;**135**:76-80

[11] Delank KW. Olfactory sensitivity in adenoid hyperplasia. Laryngo- Rhino-Otologie. 1992;**71**:293-297

[12] Suzuki M, Watanabe T, Mogi G. Clinical, bacteriological and histological study of adenoids in children. American Journal of Otolaryngology. 1999;**20**:85-90

[13] Brook I, Shah K, Jackson W. Microbiology of healthy and diseased adenoids. Laryngoscope. 2000;**110**:994-999

[14] Yasan H, Dogru H, Tuz M, et al. Otitis media with effusion and histopathologic properties of adenoid tissue. International Journal of Pediatric Otorhinolaryngology. 2003;**67**:1179-1183

[15] Shin KS, Cho SH, Kim KR, et al. The role of the adenoids in pediatric rhinosinusitis. International Journal of Pediatric Otorhinolaryngology. 2008;**72**:1643-1650

[16] Tilford DL. Unsuspected non-Hodgkins lymphoma of the tonsils and adenoids in children. Pediatrics. 1987;**79**:399-402

[17] Chohan A, Lal A, Chohan K, et al. Systematic review and meta-analysis of randomized controlled trials on the role

of mometasone in adenoid hypertrophy in children. International Journal of Pediatric Otorhinolaryngology. 2015;**79**(10):1599-1608

[18] Shin JH, Kim BG, Kim BY, Kim SW, Kim SW, Kim H. Is there an association between vitamin D deficiency and adenotonsillar hypertrophy in children with sleep-disordered breathing? BMC Pediatrics. 2018;**18**(1):196. DOI: 10.1186/s12887-018-1178-8

[19] Crowe SJ, Baylor JW. The prevention of deafness. JAMA. 1939;**112**:585-590

[20] Meyer W. On adenoid Vegetations in the Naso-pharyngeal cavity: Their pathology, diagnosis, and treatment. Med Chir Trans. 1870;**53**:191-216

[21] Weir N. Otolaryngology--an Illustrated History. Boston: MA, Butterworths; 1990

[22] Feldmann H. The nasopharynx and pharyngeal tonsil in the history of otology and rhinology. Pictures from the history of otorhinolaryngology, presented by instruments from the collection of the Ingolstadt medical history museum. Laryngorhinootologi. 1999;**78**(5):280-289

[23] Dilesh M, Adenoidectomy- A. Historical Review. Glob J Oto. 2017;**8**(3):555740. DOI: 10.19080/GJO.2017.08.555740

[24] Cannon CR, Replogle WH, Schenk MP. Endoscopic-assisted adenoidectomy. Otolaryngology-Head and Neck Surgery. 1999;**121**(6):740-744

[25] Buchinsky FJ, Lowry MA, Isaacson G. Do adenoids regrow after excision? Otolaryngology-Head and Neck Surgery. 2000;**123**(5):576-581

[26] Elluru RG, Johnson L, Myer CM. Electrocautery adenoidectomy compared with curettage and power-assisted methods. Laryngoscope. 2002;**112**(8) Pt. 2 Suppl. 100:23-25

[27] Havas T, Lowinger D. Obstructive adenoid tissue: An indication for powered shaver adenoidectomy. Archives of Otolaryngology-Head and Neck Surgery. 2002;**128**(7):789-791

[28] Stanislaw P, Koltai PJ, Feustel PJ. Comparison of power-assisted adenoidectomy vs adenoid curette adenoidectomy. Archives of Otolaryngology-Head and Neck Surgery. 2000;**126**(7):845-849

[29] Ark N, Kurtaran H, Ugur KS, Yilmaz T, Ozboduroglu AA, Mutlu C. Comparison of adenoidectomy methods: Examining with digital palpation vs. visualizing the placement of the curette. International Journal of Pediatric Otorhinolaryngology. 2010;**74**(6):649-651

[30] Koltai PJ, Chan J, Younes A. Power-assisted adenoidectomy: Total and partial resection. Laryngoscope. 2002;**112**(8) Pt. 2 Suppl. 100:29-31

[31] Rodriguez K, Murray N, Guarisco JL. Power-assisted partial adenoidectomy. Laryngoscope. 2002;**112**(8) Pt. 2 Suppl. 100:26-28

[32] Walker P. Pediatric Adenoidectomy under vision using suction-diathermy ablation. Laryngoscope. 2001;**111**(12):2173-2177

[33] Martinez SA, Akin DP. Laser tonsillectomy and adenoidectomy. Otolaryngologic Clinics of North America. 1987;**20**:371-376

[34] Wan YM, Wong KC, Ma KH. Endoscopic-guided adenoidectomy using a classic adenoid curette: A simple way

to improve adenoidectomy. Hong Kong Medical Journal. 2005;**11**(1):42-44

[35] Lo S, Rowe-Jones J. How we do it: Transoral suction diathermy adenoid ablation under direct vision using a 45 degree endoscope. Clinical Otolaryngology. 2006;**31**(5):436-455

[36] Al-Mazrou KA, Al-Qahtani A, Al-Fayez AI. Effectiveness of transnasal endoscopic powered adenoidectomy in patients with choanal adenoids. International Journal of Pediatric Otorhinolaryngology. 2009;**73**(12):1650-1652

[37] Costantini F, Salamanca F, Amaina T, Zibordi F. Videoendoscopic adenoidectomy with microdebrider. Acta Otorhinolaryngologica Italica. 2008;**28**(1):26-29

Chapter 4

3D Exoscopic Surgery (3Des) for Tonsillectomy

Sebastiano Bucolo, Matteo Pezzoli, Maria Vittoria Pomara, Umberto Visentin and Gianni Succo

Abstract

Recently we have coined the term 3Des (3D exoscopic surgery) to describe the use of the 3D Vitom Exoscope System for transoral surgery of oropharyngeal cancers. This surgical approach can also be employed for tonsillectomy performed for obstructive sleep apnea and recurrent tonsillitis. Decreasing pain, maintaining hydration, and minimizing the risk of post-operative hemorrhage has brought attention to novel surgical technique and instrumentation. The search for the most cost-effective, safe, and efficient modality that provides the maximum relief while minimizing morbidity is still ongoing. During the period from January 2022 to May 2022, 8 patients with recurrent tonsillitis were treated by tonsillectomy with the 3Des approach at our center. A comfortable transoral exposure of the tonsillar fossa and the excellent space to move the surgical instruments are the best features of this procedure, along with the great utility in the learning process, especially for residents, fellows, students.

Keywords: exoscopic surgery, 3D, tonsillectomy, video telescope operating microscopy 3D, otorhinolaryngology

1. Introduction

In the last 3 years, some studies in the ENT literature have highlighted the emerging role of exoscopes with 3D technology mainly using the VITOM [1–4]. The increasing application of 3D exoscopic technology worldwide is becoming remarkable. Exoscopic surgeries maintain the same safety profiles as those using previous surgical techniques and allow ENT surgeons to achieve better vision and illumination of small anatomic structures. In order to evaluate the exoscope potential in visualization, magnification, and dissection of deeper structures in the oral cavity we applied the 3D Vitom Exoscope System for tonsillectomy.

2. History of tonsillectomy from literature review

Tonsillectomy is one of the most commonly performed surgical procedures worldwide and since the original description of tonsillar tissue removal by Cornelius

Celsus in the First century AD, a lot of tonsillectomy techniques have been performed to decrease complications and post-operative morbidity.

The uvulotomy performed in the sixteenth century for the treatment of acute catarrhal inflammation can be considered the forerunner of tonsillectomy. This procedure inspired the scientists of the time to design suitable tools for tonsillectomy that were able to remove tonsils with a method that involved as few steps as possible to reduce complications such as the dreaded hemorrhage.

The first instrument so consisted of a metal wire which allowed the removal of the tonsil by strangulation of it. However, the operation was technically complex, took a long time, needed the management of copious bleeding, and allowed only partial excision of the tonsil which, in most cases, grew back causing recurrence. For this reason, it was during the nineteenth century that increasingly sophisticated instruments were developed to remove all the tonsil tissue in a single step. To the famous Greenfield Sluder (Washington, 1865–1928) we must give the honor of the invention of the guillotine technique made by a futuristic instrument very similar to the uvulotome used ages ago, that drastically changed the fate of patients. According to this procedure, the tonsil, placed inside the instrument, is excised from the base through a guillotine blade actioned by the surgeon. It became very famous at that time (and it's still largely used in some centers) because it was quick, almost painless, and easy both for the surgeon and for the patient, and last but not least, it responded to the knowledge and anesthesiological availability of the time. The Guillotine excision also known as the Sluder technique, despite many advantages, reported also disadvantages such as the lack of control of blood loss, a not residual tonsil tissue, accidental uvulectomy, partial accidental glossectomy, and pillar damage, as well as blood aspiration into the lower respiratory trees [5].

Soon it became clear that surgeons must look for a more anatomical and systematic approach to tonsillectomy. It's in this background that Samuel Crowe, Director of the Department of Otolaryngology at Johns Hopkins Hospital in Baltimore, stood out. Between 1911 and 1917, he performed 1000 operations with a new method and a much more cautious approach to the patient, which would inevitably revolutionize the surgical procedure: the patient was hospitalized and in the preoperative period he underwent blood tests (until then the tonsillectomy was performed during the day, without preoperative tests) and a "sharp dissection" with a scalpel was performed [6]. Above all, the position of the patient was revolutionary, with the bottom of the operating bed lower, the anesthetic gas administered through a mask, and the patient's mouth kept open with an instrument that took its name from the same surgeon (Crowe-Davis mouth gag) with the property of keeping the tongue retracted and motionless; the hemostasis is accurate and all the hemorrhagic points tied with black suture and finally, in the post-operative period the patient is not discharged until any complications are resolved.

Ideally, tonsillectomy should be a procedure that is as fast as possible, bloodless, painless, and susceptible to prompt recovery. Post-operative pain after tonsillectomy is one of the most important causes of morbidity restricting oral intake, causing dehydration and daily activity limitation [7]. In addition, restriction of the pharyngeal muscle activity due to pain, leads to a reduction in the clearance of the tonsil bed and, as a consequence of this, to infection and bleeding [8]. In 2009, some Authors [9] systematically analyzed the usefulness of the literature of the past 20 years concerning tonsillectomy technique in children and found deficits in the precise reporting of surgical techniques, adequate study design, and useful outcome measures, all of which making the literature less useful than it could be. According to the Author, the recent advances in technology, with aggressive marketing both to physicians and patients, have created additional dilemmas in clinical decision-making as far as which method of tonsillectomy will best serve the patient is concerned. As a consequence of this, many Authors suggested guidelines for studying design parameters which could lead to more valuable information for the clinician to choose the best technique for the patients.

Nowadays, the main classification of surgical tonsillectomy by dissection divides conventional and cold techniques from new hot techniques. The former includes the cold knife technique, cold dissection, sharp dissection, steel dissection, blunt dissection, snare tonsillectomy, and dissection-ligation technique. The latter, include monopolar or bipolar diathermy tonsillectomy, laser dissection (mainly represented by CO2 laser, ultrasonic dissection, radiofrequency tonsil ablation (coblation and ligasure tonsillectomy) and microdebrider tonsillectomy. In the matter in question, hot techniques, improving hemostasis, have soon replaced cold dissection techniques for most surgeons. They combine the possibility of performing cut and coagulation simultaneously taking advantage of the use of the most recent technological innovations. Due to their diffusion, versatility, and contained cost, the monopolar and bipolar electrodissections are the most used tools in tonsillectomy operations worldwide.

As far as the monopolar electrodissection is concerned, the current technical characteristics of monopolar electrodissection were instead developed simultaneously by Hall and Mann in 1984. According to them, the operation is carried out with flat-tip or sharp-tip electrosurgical units, maintaining an intensity equal to slightly higher than 20 watts (the range can however vary from 10 to 40 watts) [10]. This technique results in greater dissection precision and less intraoperative bleeding. It's perhaps the most widely used variety of tonsillectomy, so much so that in 2003 it was described by Kay and Koltai as probably the most popular method in the USA, above all due to the advantage of the short duration of the procedure and, indeed, the minimum losses intraoperative blood pressure [11] as well as for the variety of its operative tips.

It should be kept in mind that monopolar diathermy acts at a very high temperature, equal to or higher than 400°C 35, splitting the tissues thanks to the use of a radiofrequency electric current, which is transferred directly from the electrode to the tissue [12]. Similarly to bipolar and laser electrosurgery, it allows cutting and hemostasis at the same time, through overheating of the tissues generated by the resistance they oppose to the passage of the current. The heat is then able to cause cell rupture, due to a drying phenomenon, and to form a clot that obliterates the small vessels, through protein denaturation [13].

Depending on the wattage adopted (as mentioned, a power close to 20 watts is suggested), the dispersion of energy in the tissues is considerable, in particular, due to the distance between the operating electrode and the dispersive "grounding" pad. The result is large lateral damage. As a consequence of this, post-operative pain and even deferred hemorrhage episodes constitute a problem for this technique that should not be underestimated [14]. However, these aspects were not confirmed by studies by some surgeons thanks to the use of Erbe electrosurgery generator (ERBE USA). This device, contrary to what occurs in conventional systems, is characterized by the production of current at constant voltage and variable power. It is placed in theory in an intermediate position between monopolar and bipolar diathermy and can coagulate causing less thermal damage, compared to traditional monopolar electrosurgery [15].

In the study they conducted, the authors observed in particular, in the Erbe group compared to the control group, a significant reduction in pain symptoms, which was however associated with greater intraoperative bleeding and prolongation of surgical times. The application of bipolar diathermy to tonsillectomy started in the 1990s.

Initially used only for the control of hemostasis but in 1994 it was proposed as a true method of dissection. In Pang's original presentation, straight pincers with fine points were used, with the intensity of the current regulated at 30 watts [16]. Once the correct peritonsillar cleavage plane has been identified, we proceed with a practically bloodless dissection with the possibility of identifying and coagulating in a preventive and focused way most of the blood vessels afferent to the tonsil.

The introduction of bipolar electrodissection made it possible to reduce the intensity of post-operative pain, compared to the monopolar variety, thanks to the coagulation precision of the diathermic clamp, which, by transferring energy to a very limited surface, as it is included between two proximally coupled electrodes, can minimize the depth of tissue thermal damage [17]. Compared to the "hot" monopolar technique, the operation takes longer, also due to the frequent need to clean the tips of the forceps.

This drawback can be partially overcome with the use of special non-adhesive (non-stick) pliers in nickel. In bipolar diathermy, direct contact between electrodes and tissue produces a local temperature generally between 150 and 400°C, with overheating of the cellular content and consequent cellular vaporization. As regards the intensity of post-operative pain, from the investigation by Silveira et al. [18] a statistically insignificant increase emerged, particularly after the 3rd day.

In recent years, intracapsular tonsillectomy has been proposed as an alternative technique to total tonsillectomy. It consists of the resection of all the extra-velic portion of the tonsil which protrudes from the lodge: in practice, the operation will involve a drastic and progressive leveling of the profile of the tonsillar parenchyma, up to the free edge of the palatine pillars. The reason for this rediscovered interest about it is that, by preserving the tonsil capsule, it is possible to reduce post-operative pain significantly if we compare it to conventional tonsillectomy.

It can be performed with many methods such as laser, monopolar diathermy with flat tip electrode, ultrasound scalpel, plasma scalpel, and microdebrider but since it's reserved only for cases of obstructive tonsillar hypertrophy with sleep apnea, the discussion about intracapsular tonsillectomy goes beyond the aim of this chapter and will be debate elsewhere.

3. Indications and contraindications

Tonsillectomy was widely practiced in the western world as a procedure to cure a vast range of conditions from respiratory tract infections to chronic systemic diseases throughout the twentieth century [19].

In our time, the indiscriminate use of tonsillectomy that was made in past years has diminished. This was due to an increased awareness of the natural history of pharyngotonsillar infections which, together with the use of targeted antibiotic therapy and the development of specific immunomodulatory therapies, led to the creation of sophisticated and shared guidelines among ENT specialists and pediatricians.

According to clinical practice guidelines developed by the American Academy of Otolaryngology—Head and Neck Surgery Foundation and the last Italian Guidelines written in the document "Clinical and organizational appropriateness of tonsillectomy and/or adenoidectomy operations" **the indications** of tonsillectomy are recommended as follows:

1. **Airway Obstruction**

    i. Obstructive sleep apnea,

    ii. Feeding problems,

    iii. Hypernasal speech secondary to enlarged tonsils.

2. **Infections**

    i. Recurrent tonsillitis,

    ii. Peritonsillar abscess,

    iii. PFAPA (Periodic Fever, Aphthous stomatitis, Pharyngitis and cervical Adenitis) syndrome.

3. **Others**

    i. Asymmetric enlargement with suspicious of neoplasm.

Main **contraindications** are:

1. **Acute tonsillitis**: Acute infectious pathology of the tonsils or upper respiratory tract may cause an increased risk of bleeding or surgery-related pulmonary complications.

2. **Age**: Tonsillectomy is not recommended before 5 years of age for:

    i. Immune functions of the tonsils

    ii. Risk of surgery-related hypovolemic shock

3. **Anemia and bleeding diathesis**

4. Patients and procedures

We report our preliminary results on eight tonsillectomies performed between 06 January 2022 and 31 May 2022 non-consecutively at a single ENT Department using the 3Des approach (San Giovanni Bosco Hospital ENT Department, Turin).

The median patient's age was 21 years (15–28 years).

The gender distribution was 5 females vs. 3 males.

There were no exclusion criteria.

The patient cohort shows a history of recurrent tonsillitis in all cases and a history of drainages of parapharyngeal abscesses in three cases.

All the 8 operated patients had undergone previous antibiotic treatment for their disease for various exacerbations.

Three had undergone one or more parapharyngeal abscesses drainages (**Table 1**) under local anesthesia.

The procedure was performed under general anesthesia by nasopharyngeal intubation.

The patient was placed in the supine position without any interscapular support.

The mouth was held open using a Boyle Davis mouth opener.

The VITOMR 90°, mounted on a mechanical support and fixed to the operating table between 25 and 50 cm from the operating field, was connected to a camera and a light cable, while the 3D monitor(s) (which could be single or multiple) were positioned in front of the operators (**Figure 1**).

The second operator was positioned to the left or right of the first one depending on the side of the lesion, while the scrub nurse and the various trainees were positioned behind the first operator (**Figure 2**).

This setting allows everyone to follow carefully the procedure, looking at the surgical field projected onto the 3D monitor (**Figure 3**) .

Trainees can follow step by step the procedure, then they can try to perform the procedure under constant supervision by a senior surgeon, who could follow the trainees step by step thanks to the exoscopic view.

The excision was performed using the electrocautery (Force TriVerse Electrosurgical Device, Covidien, Dublin, Ireland).

The electrical current creates a temperature from 400 to 600°C allowing dissection with minimal intraoperative bleeding.

5. Results

Sixteen tonsillectomies were assessed in 8 patients from 15 to 28 years of age. Of the patients, 5 (62.5%) were female and 3 (37.5%) were male. The mean age of the patients was 20.87 (min–max: 21–36).

There was no significant occurrence of post-operative complications including post-operative fever, voice changes, ear and neck pain, immediate or delayed hemorrhage, and suture placement. Three patients reported post-operative bleeding, with a minimal amount of blood, and had spontaneous resolution with no intervention. No patient required to return to the operative room for delayed bleeding. No residual tissue was seen in any of the patients (**Table 2**).

The mean operation calculated as the time from the mouth gag to removal was 23 ± 5.6 minutes.

Age (median 21 years)	**28** ♀	**25** ♂	**16** ♀	**18** ♂	**21** ♀	**15** ♀	**23** ♀
Female	*		*		*	*	*
Male		*		*			
Recurrent infection	*	*	*	*	*	*	*
Previous parapharyngeal abscesses drainages	* (1)		*(2)				*(3)

Table 1.
Tonsillectomy group demographics.

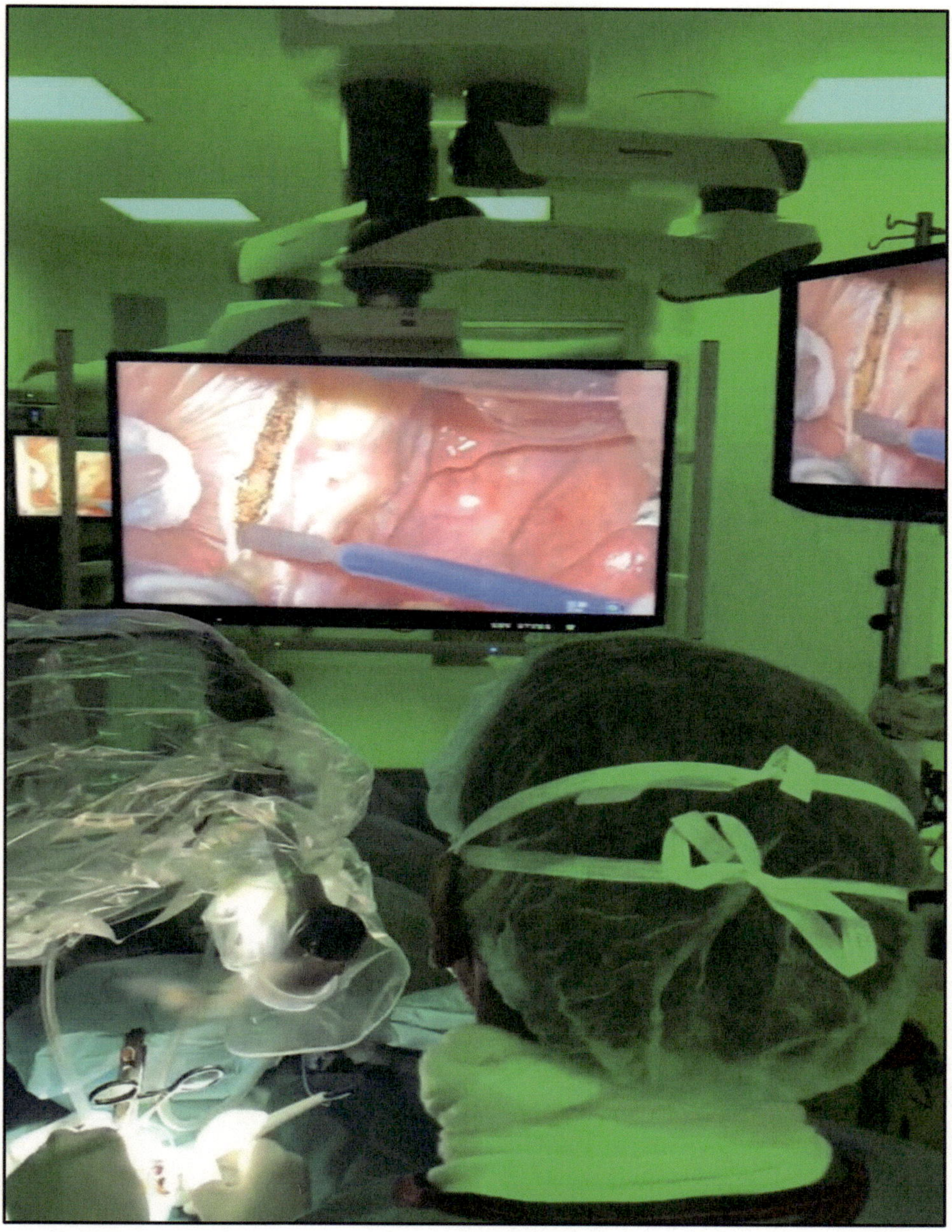

Figure 1.
3D monitor position.

No preoperative and/or post-operative anesthetic or analgesic drugs were injected into the tonsils. Patients were kept in the hospital for 24 hours for post-operation observation; all patients were discharged with stable vital signs and provided oral feeding. Patients were questioned for pain on post-operative day 1 and all the patients were discharged on post-operative day 1.

Outpatient follow-up included one visit every week for the first month. During the visit, we investigated the presence of bleeding episodes, the pain degree, and

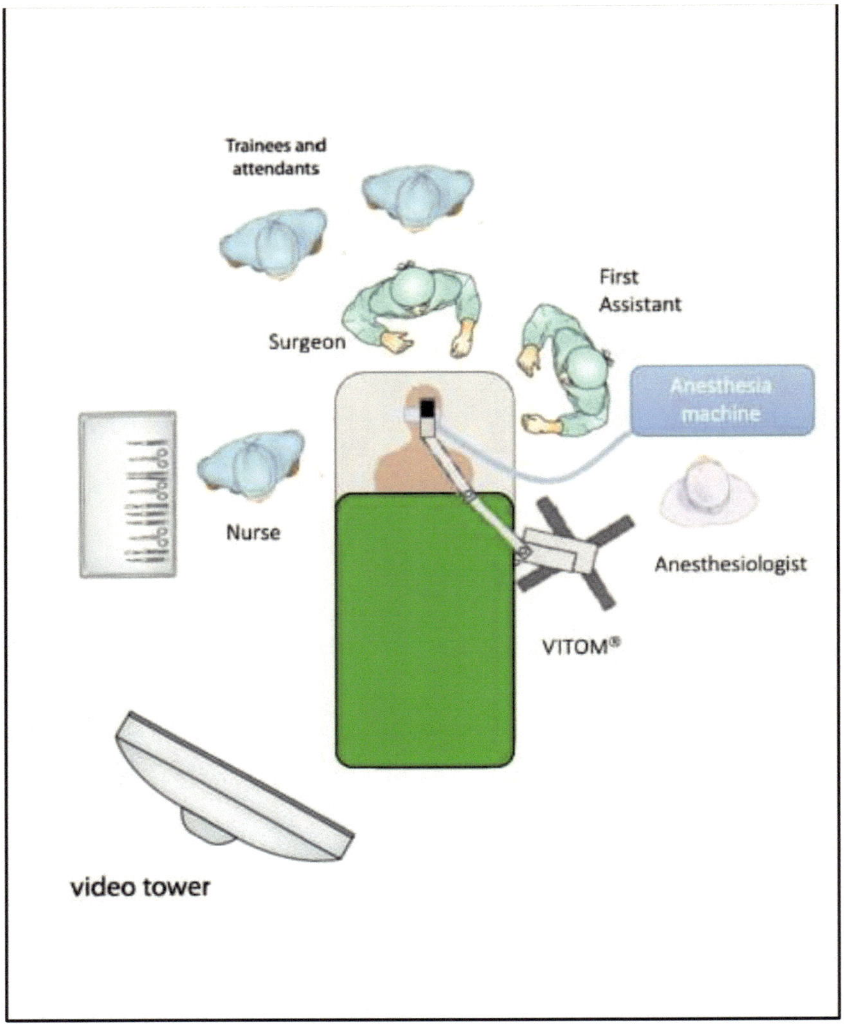

Figure 2.
Operating room setting (VITOM® Exoscope).

nutrition. All patients reported excellent subjective well-being, no bleeding episodes, and slight pain when feeding in the first two weeks.

On every visit, we performed an oropharyngeal examination through which we observed a regular fibrin formation at the tonsillectomy site.

6. Discussion

Optimal vision and ergonomics are important factors contributing to the achievement of good results during transoral surgery. Everyone knows the surgical difficulty of this district in the past when two surgeons had to working together in a narrow space, made even tighter by the presence of anesthesia equipment and with limited lighting possibilities.

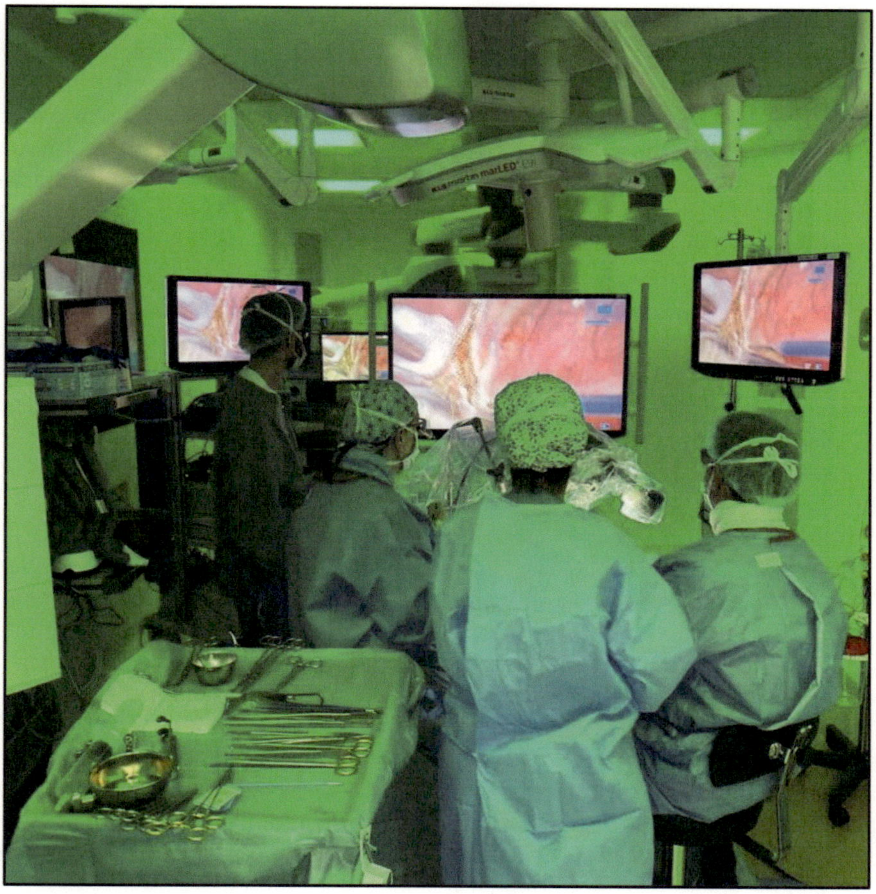

Figure 3.
Surgical team looking at the surgical field projected onto 3D monitor.

Age (median 21 years)	**28** ♀	**25** ♂	**16** ♀	**18** ♂	**21** ♀	**15** ♀	**23** ♀
Voice changes							
Ear and neck pain							
Immediate hemorrhage with spontaneous resolution	*					*	*
Delayed hemorrhage							
Suture placement							

Table 2.
Results.

Modern instruments make it possible to overcome the surgical difficulties related to factors such as uncomfortable posture and poor visibility in a very difficult anatomical district such as that of the oral cavity. Naturally, all of this favors the surgical result and minimizes the dreaded complications such as hemorrhagic complications.

Nowadays transoral tonsillectomy under naked eye is the most common procedure performed. However, this procedure does not allow an enlargement of the surgical field and this entails on the one hand the persistence of an always very high risk of bleeding especially in cases of particular anatomical narrowness of the oral cavity and on the other hand the extreme difficulty for neophyte surgeons and trainees to learn the surgical technique well from the expert surgeon who is unable to share the operating field with them. To overcome these problems, the robotic technique TORS [20] and recently endoscopic tonsillectomy [21] have been proposed to replace conventional transoral tonsillectomy, the latter with apparent interesting benefits and low costs. On the contrary, as far as TORS is concerned, the high cost of the equipment strongly limits its use in the field of benign pathology.

As far as tonsillectomy is concerned, the operating exoscope has been recently introduced and has proven to be a promising and effective tool for transoral surgery. It is in this context we coined the term 3Des (3D exoscopic surgery) to describe the use of the 3D VITOM® Exoscope System for transoral surgery especially tonsillectomy performed for obstructive sleep apnea and recurrent tonsillitis.

VITOM is the acronym for Video Telescope Operating Microscopy 3D (VITOM®—Karl Storz GmbH, Tuttlingen, Germany). Introduced in the first decade of 2000, it is an exoscope that combines 4 K resolution view with three-dimensional technology. This device is well-known and widely employed in other surgical fields such as neurosurgery, urology, and gynecology. Its introduction in head and neck surgery is quite recent but it's reaching even greater importance over time. At the moment, it is chosen in numerous otolaryngology subspecialties, such as laryngology, otology, skull base surgery, head and neck reconstruction, and of course intraoral surgery. The exoscope consists of a high-definition (HD) or 4 K (Ultra HD) 3D video camera (0° or 90°) with optical and digital zoom integrated and a fiber optic-delivered or L.E.D. light source [22]. Zoom and, focus functions and integrated illumination can be upgradeable using a double cable and light source.

This system, being covered by a sterile sheath making it suitable to be placed proximal to the area where the surgical procedure takes place, is suspended above the surgical field with a manually actuated articulating holder or robotic arm, and it is connected to a 3D monitor (55″), with a maximum screen resolution and 16:9 image format. 3D passive-polarized glasses, with anti-fog coating, or 3D clip-on glasses, circularly polarized, are worn by all staff in the operating room (OR) to view the monitor. The combination of the VITOM® system with the 3-chip sensor technology in the camera head enables excellent image quality and optimal color rendering even in non-optimal lighting conditions. The magnification power of 8–30x is possible through the 3D camera, depending on the working distance, and the size and resolution of the monitor used, while the depth of field ranges from 7 to 44 mm, with a focal distance of 20–50 cm, allowing the surgical field to be observed and illuminated at various distances from the patient. Different directions of view are possible depending on the surgical site. For tonsillectomy, 0° is considered the best option.

A comfortable transoral exposure of the lesion is sought to visualize the lesion and its boundaries completely and to have sufficient space for moving the surgical instruments. Therefore, different types of autostatic retractors can be used. For example, Boyle Davis mouth gag, with its set of tongue depressors of varying sizes supplied along with the gag, holds the tongue thereby preventing it from falling into the surgeon's field. Long surgical instruments from 24 to 30 cm need to be used because of the depth of the structures to be reached. Different kinds of cutting instruments could be used (bipolar forceps, CO2 fiber laser, ultrasound tools), and various types of angled tools were also required.

Concurrent hemostasis shortens surgical time; however, increased delivery of energy results in increased pain and odynophagia. Additionally, because of the monopolar current applied to the patient, electrocautery may interfere with or damage pacemakers, vagal nerve stimulators, and cochlear implants.

The value of transoral surgery with the 3D exoscope appears incredible in the field of surgical education of neophyte surgeons and trainees who have the opportunity to actively participate in all the surgical steps in real time, realizing the difficulties and possible complications.

The visual accuracy allows on the one hand the minimization of the dangerous bleeding complications as the identification of the small vessels is made absolutely easy and on the other hand a better accuracy in the removal of the tonsillar parenchyma avoiding injury to the surrounding tissues and reducing painful post-surgical complications.

The 3D exoscope provides surgeons with a feasible and potentially excellent alternative to traditional operating microscopes and endoscopes in head and neck surgery. Producing a high-quality video of small surgical fields, with high magnification capacity and a large depth of field, allows working in a setting that is similar to endoscopic surgeries but, unlike endoscopes, the 3D exoscope allows you to appreciate the depth and volume of anatomical structures and has a greater focal distance with a wider working space and the possibility of easy adjustment of vision. The VITOM 3D, given its excellent ability to provide three-dimensional images, depth of field, quality, and fidelity of the color and contrast of the image, is competitive in the 3D visualization of the operating field with the da Vinci robotic platform.

At present, the main disadvantages of the exoscope are represented by the mechanics of the supporting arm (it is not always comfortable to move during surgery) and the need to wear 3D glasses for a long period. Although tonsillectomies remain one of the most commonly performed surgeries in otorhinolaryngology, there is an absence of universal agreement on the surgical method and extent of removal [2]. The potential for significant morbidity, even death is inherent in the procedure. The operating exoscope with a digital camera system provides a high-definition image of the surgical field projected in a three-dimensional (3D) high-definition monitor. It allows the surgical team to operate by visualizing the magnified image of the surgical field on a screen. Recently we have coined the term 3Des (3D exoscopic surgery) to describe the use of the 3D Vitom Exoscope System for transoral surgery of oropharyngeal cancers. This surgical approach can also be employed for tonsillectomy. We performed eight tonsillectomies using this surgical approach. All the surgical steps were performed using the VITOM 3D exoscope.

The term 3Des (3D exoscopic surgery) was coined to describe the technique used for transoral surgery with the exoscope system as visual tool. The use of the exoscope enhanced the visualization of the oral cavity, thus facilitating the effectiveness of obtaining adequate surgical spaces avoiding damage to contiguous anatomical structures and giving the surgeons the possibility to maintain a more ergonomic posture [23]. The surgeon can choose to stay in a sitting or standing position, having the screen in front at the same height: the screen is placed frontally, and at the same height as the operators' eyes. This system ensures also an extensive surgical field visualization by the second surgeon and the best coordination between surgeons and nurses. Indeed, in the conventional approach, a possible disadvantage of the procedures was related to the poor precision of the second surgeon's movements due to the reduced visibility of the operating field. The same extensive surgical field visualization is enjoyed by fellows, students, and residents who want to learn this surgical technique and by the operating room staff [3]. The VITOM 3D approach allows excessively accurate hemostasis, and very precise identification of anatomical structures like the anterior and posterior tonsillar pillars, the uvula, and the palatal muscle planes.

7. Conclusions

Tonsillectomy is a surgical procedure that can be performed with multiple techniques, none of which has been recognized as the best. Nowadays transoral tonsillectomy without magnification represents the standard of care worldwide.

However, due to the advancement of technology, new procedures are being used, such as the operating exoscope. The operating exoscope has recently been introduced in various surgical specialties. In otorhinolaryngology, it has been introduced in numerous subspecialties such as laryngology, head and neck reconstructive surgery, otology, and skull base [4].

In tonsillectomy and more generally for transoral surgery, the introduction of the 3D exoscope into the surgical equipment can be of great interest for several reasons. First of all, the surgeon can operate with more precision. The exoscope magnifies the surgical image on a display and the surgeon can clearly identify all the anatomical structures of the operating field. In this way the surgeon can remove the tonsillar tissue without damaging the adjacent muscles or palatal pillars, reducing the possibility of post-operative pain. Furthermore, this allows precise identification of small vessels and accurate hemostasis, reducing the risk of intraoperative and post-operative bleeding. Furthermore, the exoscope has the advantage of standing at a distance of 20–50 cm from the patient, while the endoscope must be positioned inside the patient's mouth, limiting the surgical space.

Another invaluable advantage of the 3D exoscope is the possibility to use it for educational purposes. The first surgeon can share the operating field with all the operating room members. The surgeon can explain the procedure step-by-step, and the trainees can follow the procedure projected on the screen. During active surgical training, the use of the exoscope allows the surgeon to continuously monitor the resident without interruptions or changes of position.

The exoscopic technology also allows the surgeon to maintain a comfortable position, avoiding positions that can potentially cause muscle pain.

However, this technique also has disadvantages. First of all, during direct transoral procedures, it is difficult for the first surgeon to share the view of the surgical field with the assistants, because the exoscope instrumentation reduces the field of view. Then the lack of magnification of the surgical field may result in an imprecise visualization of the anatomical structures and hemostasis, and thus a higher risk of post-operative bleeding.

In conclusion, the use of a 3D exoscope for tonsillectomy is a valid alternative to the conventional transoral procedure. This technology offers many surgical and educational improvements and represents a major advance in one of the most common surgical procedures in otolaryngology. This technology is new and requires more retrospective or even prospective studies to investigate its superiority [24].

DOI: http://dx.doi.org/10.5772/intechopen.1001118

Acknowledgements

We would like to thank the nursing and care staff of both the recovery and the operating room.

Conflict of interest

"The authors declare no conflict of interest."

Author details

Sebastiano Bucolo*, Matteo Pezzoli, Maria Vittoria Pomara, Umberto Visentin and Gianni Succo
San Giovanni Bosco Hospital, Turin, Italy

*Address all correspondence to: sicseba@yahoo.it

References

[1] Crosetti E, Arrigoni G, Manca A, et al. 3D Exoscopic surgery (3Des) for transoral oropharyngectomy. Frontiers in Oncology. 2020;**10**:1-8

[2] De Virgilio A, Costantino A, Ms TM, Conti V, Pirola F, Russo E, et al. Pre-clinical experience with the VITOM 3D and the ARTip cruise system for Micro-laryngeal surgery. The Laryngoscope. 2021;**131**:136-138

[3] Ferlito S, La Mantia I, Caruso S, Cammaroto G, Chiesa-Estomba CM, Iannella G, et al. High definition three-dimensional exoscope (VITOM 3D) in E.N.T. surgery: A systematic review of current experience. Journal of Clinical Medicine. 2022;**11**(13):36-39

[4] Pirola F, Leone F, Di Bari M, Salamanca F, Bianchi A, Catalani M, et al. 3D 4K exoscope in snore surgery simulation: Pre-clinical experience. Sleep & Breathing. 2022. DOI: 10.1007/s11325-022-02684-1. Epub

[5] Crowe SJ, Watkins SS, Rotholz AS. Relation of tonsillar and naso-pharyngeal infections to general systemic disorders. Bulletin of the Johns Hopkins Hospital. 1917;**28**:1-25

[6] Polites N, Joniau S, Wabnitz D, Fassina R, Smythe C, Varley P, et al. Postoperative pain following coblation tonsillectomy: Randomized clinical trial. ANZ Journal of Surgery. 2006;**76**(4):226-229

[7] Belloso A, Morar P, Tahery J, Saravanan K, Nigam A, Timms MS. Randomized-controlled study comparing post-operative pain between coblation palatoplasty and laser palatoplasty. Clinical Otolaryngology. 2006;**31**(2):138-143

[8] Mink JW. Shaha S S, Brodsky L making sense out of the tonsillectomy literature. International Journal of Pediatric Otorhinolaryngology. 2009;**73**:1499-1506

[9] Maddern BR. Electrosurgery for tonsillectomy. Laryngoscope. 2002;**2**(suppl):11-13

[10] Weimert TA, Babyak JW, Richter HJ. Electrodissection tonsillectomy. Archives of Otolaryngology – Head & Neck Surgery. 1990;**116**:186-188

[11] Shah U, Galinkin J, Chiavacci R, Briggs M. Tonsillectomy by means of plasma-mediated ablation. Archives of Otolaryngology – Head & Neck Surgery. 2002;**128**:672-676

[12] Raut VV, Bhat N, Sinnathuray AR, Kinsella JB, Stevenson M, Toner JG. Bipolar scissors versus cold dissection for pediatric tonsillectomy: A prospective, randomized pilot study. International Journal of Pediatric Otorhinolaryngology. 2002;**64**:9-15

[13] Tay HL. Post-operative morbidity in electrodissection tonsillectomy. The Journal of Laryngology and Otology. 1995;**109**:209-211

[14] Neumann AM Jr, Wiatrak BJ. Erbe constant voltage electrocautery versus conventional variable voltage electrocautery for tonsillectomy in children. International Journal of Pediatric Otorhinolaryngology. 1997;**40**:35-40

[15] Pang YT, El-Hakim H, Rothera MP. Bipolar diathermy tonsillectomy. Clinical Otolaryngology. 1994;**19**:355-357

[16] Sheahan P, Miller I, Colreavy M, Sheahan JN, McShane D, Curran A. The

ultrasonically activated scalpel versus bipolar diathermy for tonsillectomy: A prospective, randomized trial. Clinical Otolaryngology. 2004;**29**:530-534

[17] Silveira H, Silveira Soares J, Almeida LH. Tonsillectomy: Cold dissection versus bipolar electrodissection. International Journal of Pediatric Otorhinolaryngology. 2003;**67**:345-351

[18] Kornblut AD. A traditional approach to surgery of the tonsils and adenoids. Otolaryngological Clinic North America. 1987;**20**:249-263

[19] Younis RT, Lazar RH. History and current practice of tonsillectomy. The Laryngoscope. 2002;**112**(Suppl):3-5

[20] Weinstein GS, Quon H, Newman HJ, et al. Transoral robotic surgery alone for oropharyngeal cancer: An analysis of local control. Archives of Otolaryngology - Head and Neck Surgery. 2012;**138**(7):628-634

[21] Nakaya M, Kimura Y, Onuki Y, et al. Endoscopic-assisted tonsillectomy. Laryngoscope. 2013;**123**:360-361

[22] Colombo G, Ferreli F, Di Bari M, Cugini G, Miceli S, De Virgilio A, et al. Introducing the high-definition 3D exoscope in ear surgery: Preliminary analysis of advantages and limits compared with operative microscope. European Archives of Oto-Rhino-Laryngology. 2021;**278**:4217-4223. DOI: 10.1007/s00405-020-06510-w

[23] Ridge SE, Shetty KR, Lee DJ. Heads-up surgery: Endoscopes and exoscopes for otology and Neurotology in the era of the COVID-19 pandemic. Otolaryngologic Clinics of North America. 2021;**54**:11-23

[24] Festa BM, Zuppardo J, Costantino A, Ferreli F, Spriano G, Mercante G, et al. High-definition 3D exoscope-assisted tonsillectomy. American Journal of Otolaryngology. 2023;**44**(1):103674. DOI: 10.1016/j.amjoto.2022.103674

Chapter 5

The Link between Adenoids and Nasopharyngeal Carcinoma

Du-Bois Asante, Patrick Kafui Akakpo and Gideon Akuamoah Wiafe

Abstract

Adenoids, play a significant role in inflammatory response, especially in children. Together with other tissues of the lymphatic system, it fights off infections. In most cases of nasopharyngeal cancer, though rare, other histopathological variants of adenoids are seen. Adenoid hypertrophy is mostly observed, which causes obstruction of the nasopharynx and dysfunction of the Eustachian tube because of the formation of an abnormal tissue mass. Different viral and bacterial pathogens are associated with adenoid hypertrophy, including Epstein-Barr virus (EBV), coronavirus, parainfluenza virus, *Mycoplasma pneumoniae*, *Staphylococcus aureus*, and *Neisseria gonorrhoeae*. Among these, EBV is associated with both adenoid hypertrophy and nasopharyngeal cancer, indicating the effect of EBV on both nasopharyngeal cancer and adenoids. We critically appraise the current evidence and discuss potential link between adenoids and nasopharyngeal carcinoma.

Keywords: adenoids, nasopharyngeal carcinoma, Epstein-Barr virus, adenoid hypertrophy, nasopharynx, lymphoid tissue

1. Introduction

Adenoids also known as nasopharyngeal tonsils, is a collection of lymphoid tissue found on the level of the soft palate, at the posterior wall of the nasopharynx. At this site, the introduction of antigens through the nasal and oral cavities, are detected by the lymphocytes in the Waldeyer's ring [1].

This results in the priming of the infant's immune system, ultimately contributing further towards immunologic memory and production of antibodies in children. Adenoids are present at birth and enlarge to a maximum size usually in children, after which adenoidal tissue atrophy occurs. They are nearly absent during adulthood. Thus, adenoiditis is commonly a disease diagnosed during childhood and adolescence. Adenoiditis or hypertrophic adenoids occurs when there is inflammation of the adenoid tissue resulting from infection, allergies, or irritation from acid chyme reflux. In adults, they may be as a result of compromised immunity. Persistence of the etiological agents may lead to adenoid hypertrophy, which is responsible for many of the complications of adenoid disease, including Eustachian tube dysfunction and recurrent acute otitis media [2]. Malignant forms of adenoids are called adenoid cyst carcinoma, and though rare (about 1% of all carcinomas of the head and neck), they are locally aggressive and show perineural invasion [3].

Nasopharyngeal carcinoma (NPC) on the other hand, is classified as a malignant neoplasm, arising from the mucosal epithelium of the nasopharynx, most often within the lateral nasopharyngeal recess or fossa of Rosenmüller [4]. Unlike other cancer types that are primarily linked with the aged, NPC can also be seen in children [5] and young patients [6]. In South China (where NPC is an epidemic disease), hypertrophic adenoids and NPC are commonly diagnosed together, mainly in young individuals [7].

Similarly, EBV as an aetiological agent, is a commoner of both adenoids [8, 9] and NPCs [10]. Hence, due to their anatomical location, a common aetiological agent, these two lesions, in some cases are commonly diagnosed together in the ear, nose and throat (ENT) departments of hospitals and also coexist in young individuals. Differentiating these two from each other during treatment could prevent overdosage and measurement of potentially false tumour size. And this is crucial, as response to therapy by these two lesions are different [11].

In recent years, multiple studies have been carried out on adenoids and NPC separately, but few have looked at their coexistence in a patient. Thus, we carried out a literature search in NCBI PubMed using 'Adenoids' together with 'Nasopharyngeal carcinoma' as single entities or together.

We summarized the findings of these studies and discuss potential link between adenoids and nasopharyngeal carcinoma.

2. Adenoids

Adenoids develop from week 6 of gestation [12], and are described as lymphatic tissue mass lining the roof and posterior superior wall of the nasopharynx [12, 13]. Adenoids form a larger part of the lymphatic tissue of the Waldeyer's ring comprising palatine, pharyngeal and lingual tonsils. These tonsils constitute the mucosa-associated lymphoid tissue (MALT) [1, 13, 14] and specifically function as an important part of the immune system early in human life. The Waldeyer's ring is named after a twentieth-century German anatomist, Heinrich Wilhelm Gottfried von Waldeyer-Hartz. Blood supply to the adenoids is by the ascending pharyngeal artery, ascending palatine artery, the tonsillar branch of the facial artery, the pharyngeal branch of the maxillary artery, artery of the pterygoid and the basisphenoid artery. Venous drainage is via the pharyngeal venous plexuses through the paratonsillar veins to the facial and internal jugular veins. The lymphatic drainage of the adenoids is directed via the retropharyngeal and pharyngomaxillary lymph nodes [15]. Adenoids act as the first site of defense against infectious agents and inhaled allergens in the nasopharynx. With their ciliated epithelial lining, they sample pathogens and generate immune responses against them. This sometimes leads to the development of immunologic memory which persists throughout childhood.

Adenoids are relatively small at birth, grow and peak in size around age 10. They gradually atrophy in adolescents to late adulthood [16, 17]. The hypertrophy of adenoids observed in children around age 6–10 is physiologically normal. However, these hypertrophied adenoids in children and adults are commonly linked to chronic infections, and sometimes allergies [18]. Since adenoids are largely seen in children, adenoid hypertrophy (AH) is more present in children than in adults, with 34.46% prevalence in children and adolescents [19]. AH causes a blockage in the airflow through the nasopharynx forcing affected individuals to breathe through the mouth. This results in difficulties in feeding, sleeping and speech [20, 21]. Otitis media (resulting from the obstruction of the orifice of the eustachian tube), cranial facies, chronic rhinosinusitis, snoring, cough, restlessness and attention deficits are among the observed symptoms that result from AH. Hypoxia and hypercarbia are also seen in extreme cases [18, 22–24]. Persistent untreated hypertrophy of adenoids exacerbates infections and reduces immunity which may lead to the development of other infection induced complications [25]. Overall, its anatomical position in the region of the nasopharynx exposes it to many and variety of microorganisms and allergens, making it an ever-active first line immunological ground.

3. Nasopharyngeal cancer

NPC is a malignant squamous cell carcinoma that originates in the nasopharynx (specifically the pharyngeal recess, thus the fossa of Rosenmüller). Though uncommon in most part of the world, it is geographically endemic in populations of Southern China, Southeast Asia, the Artic, some parts of North Africa and the Middle-East [26–29]. Out of the 129,079 cases of NPC reported globally in 2018 by the International Agency for Research on Cancer, Asia recorded over 85% of the reported cases. Over 72,000 mortality cases were recorded with only China accounting for 40.14% [26, 30–32]. Reports indicate that NPC disproportionately affects males than females [26, 29, 33, 34]. Studies conducted in North America revealed a higher incidence of NPC among migrated Asian population as compared to resident Caucasians, suggesting a genetic predisposition to the occurrence of the carcinoma [35–37].

Histologically, the World Health Organization (WHO) classifies NPC into three major forms: type I-keratinizing squamous cell carcinoma (SCC), type II-non-keratinizing differentiated squamous cell carcinoma and type III-non-keratinizing undifferentiated squamous cell carcinoma. A rare variant, basaloid SCC has also been identified [26, 28, 37]. Type I is more common in other parts of the world whereas Type II and III are mostly seen in NPC cases from endemic areas [38].

4. Anatomical and pathological relationship between adenoids and nasopharyngeal cancer

Due to their location, both AH and NPC have the potential to cause obstruction of the orifice of the Eustachian tubes leading to serous otitis media and middle ear infections [39, 40]. This can potentially progress [41, 42] leading to hearing loss and speech problems. AH has the ability to expand into the posterior choanae and cover significant sections of the nasopharynx, obstructing airflow and causing mouth breathing [43]. In 2014, a retrospective study conducted by Berkiten et al. reported that 82.95% of (over 1600 individuals) patients had undifferentiated NPC with nasal obstruction as the common symptom. Interestingly, the study also concluded that hypertrophic adenoids are the major cause of nasal obstruction observed in these adult patients [44]. And this aforementioned condition is also common in children [45]. The abnormal inflammation of the adenoid presents an environment for the potential development of NPC since unresolved proliferation of the adenoidal lymphoid tissue reduces immunity at the nasopharyngeal region, allowing for recurrent infections as seen in EBV reported cases.

No.	Condition (NPC/ Adenoid)	Causative agent(s) identified	Histotype present	Observed symptoms	Technique used	Treatment option	Age range (years)	References
1	AH	NR	NR	NR	Lateral neck X-ray	NR	5–14	Moideen et al. [23]
2	AH	Human herpesviruses 6, cytomegalovirus, EBV	NR	NR	Quantitative real-time PCR	NR	2–11	Lomaeva et al. [47]
3	AH	NR	NR	NR	Lateral cephalogram	NR	6–11	Zhao et al. [24]
4	AH	NR	NR	NR	Lateral soft tissue neck X-ray	Adenoidectomy	2–16	Shuaibu et al. [48]
5	AH	NR	NR	NR	MRI	NR	0–82	Surov et al. [49]
6	AH	NR	NR	NR	Flexible fibreoptic endoscopy	Nasal irrigations with isotonic solution and antihistamine medications	2–14	Cassano et al. [50]
7	AH	Nasal allergy, *S. pneumoniae*	NR	Mouth breathing, bilateral nasal obstruction, snoring, headache, nasal allergy, earache, hearing loss	Flexible fibreoptic endoscopy, radiology	NR	3–14	Maheswaran et al. [51]
8	AH	NR	NR	Snoring, mouth breathing and sleep discomfort	Lateral neck radiography, nasal endoscopy	Montelukast chewable tablets	4–12	Shokouhi et al. [52]

No.	Condition (NPC/ Adenoid)	Causative agent(s) identified	Histotype present	Observed symptoms	Technique used	Treatment option	Age range (years)	References
9	AH	NR	NR	NR	Powered-shaver adenoidectomy	NR	10–14	Havas and Lowinger [43]
10	AH	NR	NR	Snoring, mouth breathing and sleep apnoea, otitis media, recurrent pharyngitis	Lateral nasopharyngeal X-ray	NR	0–15	Dixit and Tripathi [53]
11	AH	NR	NR	NR	Flexible fibreoptic nasopharynx endoscopy (FNE)	Adenoidectomy (Backmann adenotome)	3–9	Zwierz et al. [54]
12	AH	NR	NR	Snoring, sleep apnoea, mouth breathing, and otitis media	Lateral neck radiography, fibre-optic rhinoscopy	NR	NR	Mlynarek et al. [55]
13	AH	NR	NR	Snoring, mouth breathing, daytime noisy breathing, sleep apnoea	Flexible fibreoptic endoscopy	NR	2–12	Kindermann et al. [56]
14	AH	EBV	NR	NR	EBV DNA by real-time quantitative PCR	NR	2–14	Zhang et al. [57]
15	AH	Adenovirus	NR	Rhinorrhoea, otitis media	Physical examination, direct nasal endoscopy, MRI, PET	Radiotherapy	10	Nicodemo et al. [19]

No.	Condition (NPC/ Adenoid)	Causative agent(s) identified	Histotype present	Observed symptoms	Technique used	Treatment option	Age range (years)	References
16	NPC	NR	Squamous cell carcinoma, non-Hodgkins lymphoma, plasmacytoma, rhabdomyosarcoma	NR	NR	Chemotherapy, radiotherapy	14–60	Iseh et al. [33]
17	NPC	EBV	Lympho-epithelioma	NR	Immunological assessment for EBV, radiology, biopsies	Radio-chemotherapy	9–80	Bofares [58]
18	NPC	NR	Non-keratinized undifferentiated SCC	NR	^{18}F-FDG PET/MRI	NR	NR	Feng et al. [59]
19	NPC	NR	Differentiated SCC, undifferentiated SCC	NR	Computed tomography (CT)	NR	40–75	Raica et al. [60]
20	NPC	EBV	NR	NR	Endoscopy and MRI	NR	30–70	Liu et al. [61]
21	NPC	NR	NR	NR	Endoscopy and MRI	NR	17–86	Shayah et al. [62]
22	NPC	EBV	NR	NR	Serum analysis for EBV antibodies	NR	30–59	Ji et al. [63]
23	NPC	NR	NPC type I, II and III	Otitis media, hearing loss, obstruction, epistaxis, headache, neuropathy, neck mass	Endoscopy and MRI	NR	NR	Wang et al. [64]
24	NPC	EBV	Diffused symmetrical and asymmetrical hyperplasia, mucosal lesion	NR	Endoscopy and MRI	NR	40–62	King et al. [65]

No.	Condition (NPC/ Adenoid)	Causative agent(s) identified	Histotype present	Observed symptoms	Technique used	Treatment option	Age range (years)	References
25	NPC	NR	NR	NR	Endoscopy, endoscopic biopsy and MRI	NR	17–85	King et al. [66]
26	NPC	NR	Lymphoid hyperplasia	NR	Biopsy, MRI	NR	21–94	King et al. [67]
27	NPC	NR	NR	Nasal obstruction, epistaxis and hearing loss	Endoscopic biopsy, sonography and MRI	NR	21–68	Gao et al. [68]
28	NPC	EBV	NR	NR	Serum EBV capsid antigen IgA	NR	NR	Chen et al. [69]
29	NPC	NR	Non-keratinized undifferentiated SCC	NR	PET/MRI and PET/CT	NR	24–77	Cheng et al. [70]
30	NPC	NR	NR	NR	Whole-body ^{18}F-FDG PET/MRI, ^{18}F-FDG-PET/CT	Radiation therapy, chemoradiotherapy, platinum-based chemotherapy	NR	Chan et al. [71]
31	NPC	NR	Non-keratinized carcinoma	NR	Serological testing for VCA/IgA, EA/IgA, Rta/IgG and EBNA1/IgA antibodies for EBV	NR	30–70	Cai et al. [72]
32	NPC	NR	Undifferentiated NPC	Nasal obstruction and bleeding	FNE, lateral radiography, MRI, FDG-PET	Radiotherapy and chemotherapy	7	Cengiz et al. [73]

Table 1.
List of NPC and adenoid hypertrophy cases.

Similarly, unlike other cancer types that are primarily associated with the aged, NPC can also be seen in children [5, 46] and young patients [6], depicting that AH and NPC can affect both children and adults (**Table 1**). For instance, in South China (where NPC is an epidemic disease), hypertrophic adenoids and NPC are commonly diagnosed together, mainly in young individuals [7].

Overall, since both lesions arise in the nasopharynx, the co-occurrence of the two in a patient will be very crucial during diagnosis and treatment regimes. Thus, effective diagnosis of these lesions in cases where they coexist is very important.

5. Aetiological agents for AH and NPC

Myriad causative agents have been identified to contribute to the development of AH and NPC, ranging from infectious to non-infectious agents and genetic predisposition. For AH, recurrent viral and bacterial infections in the upper respiratory tract is known to be the major cause. Reported viral pathogens include adenovirus, rhinovirus, cytomegalovirus, herpes simplex virus, EBV, coronavirus, parainfluenza virus and coxsackievirus [47, 74, 75]. France et al. [76] reported the incidence of AH in human immunodeficiency virus (HIV) patients which confirmed the findings of Olsen et al. [77]. Rout et al. also suggested that the immunity of HIV patients are compromised and further reported that adults receiving organ transplants might be prone to developing AH [78]. Aerobic and non-aerobic bacterial pathogens associated with AH include *Streptococcus pneumoniae*, *Peptostreptococcus*, *Enterococcus* species, *Bacteroides*, *Streptococcus viridans*, *Streptococcus pyrogens*, *Prevotella* species, *Moraxella catarrhalis*, *Klebsiella*, *Fusobacterium*, *Staphylococcus epididermis*, *Escherichia coli* and *Haemophilus influenzae* [74, 79]. Allergies, smoking, gastroesophageal reflux and air pollution are some of the non-infectious agents that cause AH. Other factors such as sinonasal malignancy and lymphoma are also associated with AH [74, 80]. Recently, Gao et al. discovered that extracellular signal-regulated kinase 1/2 activation by cysteinyl leukotriene receptor 1 may contribute to the development of AH [81]. Similarly, NACHT LRR and PYD domains-containing protein 3 (NLRP3)-mediated pyroptosis has been shown to be a mechanism through which IL-32 influences the progression of AH [82]. Additionally, a higher chance of developing AH has also been linked to several genetic predisposing factors [83–86]. However, in a recent study conducted in Moscow, Lomaeva et al. suggested that children aged 2–11 years with the IL-10G-1082A genotype GG might be resistant to the development of AH [47].

Although the primary aetiology of NPC remains indefinite, EBV has strongly been associated with developing NPC and is mostly seen in the endemic areas, mostly associated with the type III [26, 28, 87–92]. Other infections such as human papillomavirus (HPV) has also been identified in NPC cases and found to be an aetiological agent for the development of NPC [37]. However, Bossi et al. recently reported that though HPV is highly seen in type I NPC, limited data is available on its association with NPC prognosis [93]. Among the HPV-positive/EBV-negative cases identified mostly in the non-endemic regions, worse patient outcomes have been observed than in EBV-positive cases [94].

A review by Chua et al. in 2016 indicated that persons with non-viral aetiologies of NPCs had lower survival rates and a worse phenotypic expression of the disease as compared to viral-associated causes [38]. This shows that the non-viral oncogenic variants have serious implications and yet their mechanistic mode of action remain undetermined. Reported non-viral aetiologies of NPCs include tobacco and smoking [87]. Risk of developing NPC have also been associated with alcohol intake, passive, intensity and frequency of smoking [95]. Though diet play a lesser role in the development of NPC currently [26], nitrosamines found in Chinese-styled salted fish and other preserved foods pose a high risk for the development of NPC [37]. These are associated with the non-keratinizing SCC of NPCs in the endemic regions while smoking and alcohol intake have been reported to cause type I NPCs mostly found in the non-endemic regions [37, 38]. Green-leafy vegetable diets seems to have a lower NPC risk as compared to animal based diets which has a twofold increased risk [96]. Additionally, frequent exposure to formaldehyde and wood dust are known causes of NPC [26]. However, other studies reported elsewhere found no excess risk in the development of NPC [97–100]. High risk genetic vulnerability have also been implicated in individuals with susceptibility loci on class I and II human leukocyte antigen (HLA) molecules in genome wide studies [29, 101–106]. Other reported genes of influence include cell cycle genes *MDM2* and *TP53*, cell movement/adhesion gene *MMP2* and DNA repair gene *RAD51L1* [107].

Among the reported causative agents for AH and NPC, EBV and other lifestyle activities such as smoking and air pollution are common among the two, indicating the potential effect these agents have on adenoids and the nasopharynx.

6. Techniques for diagnosis

6.1 Adenoid hypertrophy

A major issue affecting the paediatric population is diseases of ENT of which AH is no exception. Early diagnosis is therefore necessary to control symptoms and enhance treatment modalities. Zwierz et al. grouped the various diagnostic methods into two categories: namely, invasive and imaging [54]. They further grouped techniques such as rigid or flexible fibreoptic nasopharynx endoscopy (FFNE), video fluoroscopy, acoustic rhinomanometry, physical examination by the finger or a mirror through the mouth as invasive. Lateral nasopharyngeal X-ray, ultrasonography, and magnetic resonance imaging (MRI) of the nasopharynx are grouped as imaging techniques. Other imaging techniques such as computed tomography (CT) and cone beam tomography have also been reported [108]. These procedures come with high costs, the need for ENT specialists and cutting-edge expensive equipments. Though Zwierz et al. [54] reported that FFNE is invasive, Baldassari and Choi [109] highlighted that FFNE is minimally invasive and reliable among the paediatric population due to its effective and dynamic approach. Several other studies have also reported that FFNE is the gold standard for examining the nasopharynx which is less expensive as compared to the image techniques [50, 110–116]. FFNE is also the preferred choice of diagnostic procedure because it does not expose patients to unnecessary radiation as the imaging techniques do. In a recent retrospective study by Narang et al., 86% of children aged 3–10 years responded to the technique with no signs of discomfort, and symptoms of AH such as snoring, mouth-breathing and apnoeic episodes positively correlated with adenoid size [117].

Diagnosis of adenoid size in children with AH using video fluoroscopy yielded a 100% sensitivity and 90% specificity as compared to lateral skull films which showed 70% sensitivity and 55% specificity. This study concluded that video fluoroscopy is also a less invasive and reliable technique for the diagnosis of AH in the paediatric population [115]. On a lateral cephalogram ENT surgeons use methods such as that proposed by Handelman and Osborne which uses a trapezoid analysis to evaluate the adenoid-airway area [118]. Other methods have been formulated in recent years [119–121]. Among these, Choudhari and Shrivastav in a recent study, found the methods proposed by Holmberg and Linder-Aronson and Maw et al. to have better diagnostic accuracy due to their high sensitivity and specificity [108]. Adenoid-nasopharyngeal (A/N) ratio has also been used to assess adenoid size in several AH studies [23, 53, 122–125], proposed earlier by Fujioka et al. [126]. These studies used lateral X-rays/cephalograms and found a positive correlation between adenoid size and severity of AH symptoms. Consequently, they concluded that lateral X-rays can also be used in the diagnosis of adenoid hypertrophies. Contrastingly, Mlynarek et al. concluded in their study that video rhinoscopy better correlated with adenoid size than lateral neck radioscopy [55]. However, Moideen et al. suggested that when images are not clear, FFNE should be used to give a definite diagnostic evaluation of hypertrophied adenoids [23]. In a systematic review by Major et al. which focused on comparing nasoendoscopy with other various diagnostic procedures for evaluating AH by dentists, lateral cephalogram was found to be a better option when used in combination with in-depth patient medical history [127]. Intra-operative mirror exam have also been used to assess adenoid size using the A/N ratio in comparison with FFNE findings [125, 128].

6.2 Nasopharyngeal cancer

Tissue biopsy is the gold standard for definite diagnosis of NPC though it is invasive [66].

Since EBV is highly associated with the occurrence of NPC [129], circulating free plasma EBV DNA has been used as a non-invasive biomarker to screen the disease, suggest treatment options and monitor the disease prognosis and recurrence [130, 131]. This technique produced an outstanding specificity (97.1%) and sensitivity (98.6%) in a prospective study where screening was done in a large sample of Chinese asymptomatic males aged between 40 and 69 years. The study concluded that this technique is reliable in detecting early stages of NPC which is advantageous in monitoring effective treatment and preventing worse disease outcomes [130]. In a more recent meta-analysis, EBV DNA gave a higher diagnostic accuracy than its related antibodies (VC-IgA, EBNA1-IgA and Rta-IgG) [132]. Early stages of NPC which sometimes presents with asymptomatic patients can be detected with immunoglobulin A (IgA) antibodies against EBV using various enzyme-linked immunosorbent assay (ELISA) and chemiluminescent immunoassays kits [63, 69, 133, 134]. Similarly, a meta-analysis of 21 studies by Li et al. also showed that the presence of VC/IgA in NPC-positive serum is suggestive of the presence of the disease [135]. However, a combined detection of EBV capsid antigen-IgA (VC-IgA) and early lytic gene (BRLF1) transcription activator (Rta)-IgG have been reported to give better serodiagnosis of NPC than VC/IgA alone in a Southern Chinee population [72]. In 130 EBV-positive individuals who were NPC asymptomatic, 7 cases of NPC were identified when fibreoptic endoscopy was combined with biopsy in the evaluation of some sites of the nasopharynx [136].

A combined imaging technique using positron emission tomography (PET) and MRI (PET/MRI) have shown better diagnostic images than PET/CT technique [70]. A similar observation was reported [71] where images from PET/MRI were more detailed and succinct than those of PET/CT. PET/MRI therefore produced definite images that enhanced staging procedures in NPC. In a radiomic study, Feng et al. also developed a combined radiomic model based on fluorine-18 fludeoxyglucose (fFE)-PET/MRI and PET semiquantitative parameters (metabolic tumour volume, total lesion glycolysis and standardized uptake value). They concluded that this model was also reliable in the staging of NPC [59]. The use of MRI in the early stages of NPC is however not highly recommended because of its diminished sensitivity in detecting small mucosal lesions. Contrastingly, because of its remarkable sensitivity, nasopharynx MRI with gadolinium enhancement is encouraged for use in localized staging of NPC [137]. In a population study, Liu et al. compared MRI with conventional endoscopy in the detection of NPC and concluded that MRI has a better sensitivity than endoscopy [61]. Raica et al. reported that neither clinical or endoscopic examination is a clear-cut technique in detecting the extent of tumour metastasis observed in NPC. This may be because the tumours are tiny during the initial endoscopic examination [137], located in the submucosal layer [136], or present in conjunction with hyperplasia [138]. Additionally, the lateral pharyngeal recess may be structurally difficult to find due to its location which hinders a clinician's ability to identify an occult NPC [64, 139]. Raica et al. however stated in their study of 16 patients with different histologic forms of SCC which implored the use of CT and concluded that CT scan is able to predict the staging of NPC [60]. Sonography has been compared with MRI in the diagnosis of NPC among endemic population. Similar detection of cancer was observed between the two techniques in terms of sensitivity, specificity and accuracy [68]. In a parallel study where the sensitivity and specificity of ultrasonography was compared with endoscopy, similar observations were recorded in the detection of NPC [140].

In cases of NPC where AH is concurrently diagnosed, MRI is the best option to distinguish the two lesions [141, 142]. In a case report of a 7-year-old boy who presented with nasal congestion and obstruction, AH was suspected. However, further diagnosis using immunohistochemistry revealed that the histology of the tissue mass was undifferentiated NPC [73]. Thus, tissue specific antibodies can be used alongside to aid validate the initial diagnosis to prevent false results. A summary of the techniques used in the diagnosis of AH and NPC is presented in **Table 1**. Although similar diagnostic techniques have been reported for NPC and AH with promising results, it is recommended that well defined standards be established to help in the prompt diagnosis of the lesions in both endemic and non-endemic regions. This will enhance effective differential diagnosis, better prognostic measures, treatment modalities and increase survival rates among patients.

7. Treatment and future perspectives

NPC have mostly been treated using platinum based chemotherapy, radiotherapy or chemoradiotherapy [33, 71]. In the more advanced stages such as stage IVB, other options include the use of immunotherapy alone or in combination with chemotherapy [143]. Also, chemotherapy plus targeted therapy (Cetuximab) or immunotherapy may be other options used in this more advanced stage [144]. In recurrent NPC, endoscopic surgery is also done to reduce tumour load before radiotherapy. Other options include chemotherapy or immunotherapy (or both). The targeted drug cetuximab may be given along with chemotherapy. Hence, immunotherapy and targeted therapy might be the last treatment option for advanced stage or recurrent NPC. The two treatment regimens (targeted therapy and immunotherapy) have shown preliminary antitumour effects, and have acceptable adverse effects [143].

For adenoids, they are treated primarily by adenoidectomy [48, 54]. Other treatment modalities for adenoids include nasal irrigations with an isotonic solution and antihistamine medications [50] and chewing Montelukast tablets [52].

However, there are unique cases where there is co-existence of benign or hypertrophic adenoids with NPC. In such instances, these non-malignant tissues should technically not be considered as gross tumour volume (GTV) during radiotherapy. This is because, distinction of adjacent non-malignant adenoidal tissues will allow for precise measurement of GTV to avoid overdosed radiation and guide delivery of radiation to reduce non-specific toxicity in normal tissue. Furthermore, the adenoids and NPC may have different responses to chemoradiotherapy and radiotherapy [11, 142].

Lastly, the advent of liquid biopsy analysis such as circulating tumour cells (CTCs), circulating tumour DNA (ctDNA), extracellular vesicles and micro-RNAs (miRNAs) in recent years, have demonstrated the feasibility of applying these biomarkers as a prognostic and/or predictive tool in patients with NPC [145]. These methods not only determine the heterogeneity of the tumour, but can also detect mutations or markers that are potentially druggable, hence enhancing the delivery of targeted therapy for effective treatment of the disease [144, 146].

8. Conclusion

From this review, enough evidence points to the fact that both AH and NPC have a common link based on the anatomical location and pathologies. More specifically, similar symptoms and common aetiological agents are observed in both disease conditions, and prevalent in both children and adults.

Author details

Du-Bois Asante[1,2]*, Patrick Kafui Akakpo[3] and Gideon Akuamoah Wiafe[2]

1 Department of Forensic Science, University of Cape Coast, Ghana

2 Department of Biomedical Sciences, University of Cape Coast, Ghana

3 Department of Pathology, University of Cape Coast, Ghana

*Address all correspondence to: duasante@ucc.edu.gh

References

[1] Hellings P, Jorissen M, Ceuppens JL. The Waldeyer's ring. Acta Oto-Rhino-Laryngologica Belgica. 2000;**54**:237-241

[2] Schupper AJ, Nation J, Pransky S. Adenoidectomy in children: What is the evidence and what is its role? Current Otorhinolaryngology Reports. 2018;**6**:64-73. DOI: 10.1007/s40136-018-0190-8

[3] Barrett AW, Speight PM. Perineural invasion in adenoid cystic carcinoma of the salivary glands: A valid prognostic indicator? Oral Oncology. 2009;**45**:936-940. DOI: 10.1016/j.oraloncology.2009.07.001

[4] Larem A, Al Duhirat E, Omer H. Nasopharyngeal cancer. In: Al-Qahtani A, Haidar H, Larem A, editors. Textb. Clin. Otolaryngol. Cham: Springer International Publishing; 2021. pp. 479-485. DOI: 10.1007/978-3-030-54088-3_41

[5] Kao W-C, Chen J-S, Yen C-J. Advanced nasopharyngeal carcinoma in children. Journal of Cancer Research and Practice. 2016;**3**:84-88. DOI: 10.1016/j.jcrpr.2016.05.007

[6] Zhu Y, Song X, Li R, Quan H, Yan L. Assessment of nasopharyngeal cancer in young patients aged ≤ 30 years. Frontiers in Oncology. 2019;**9**:1-8. Available from: https://www.frontiersin.org/articles/10.3389/fonc.2019.01179. [Accessed: February 11, 2023]

[7] Wei K-R, Zheng R-S, Zhang S-W, Liang Z-H, Ou Z-X, Chen W-Q. Nasopharyngeal carcinoma incidence and mortality in China in 2010. Chinese Journal of Cancer. 2014;**33**:381-387. DOI: 10.5732/cjc.014.10086

[8] Al-Salam S, Dhaheri SA, Awwad A, Daoud S, Shams A, Ashari MA. Prevalence of Epstein–Barr virus in tonsils and adenoids of United Arab Emirates nationals. International Journal of Pediatric Otorhinolaryngology. 2011;**75**:1160-1166. DOI: 10.1016/j.ijporl.2011.06.012

[9] Seishima N, Kondo S, Wakisaka N, Kobayashi E, Imoto T, Moriyama-Kita M, et al. EBV infection is prevalent in the adenoid and palatine tonsils in adults. Journal of Medical Virology. 2017;**89**:1088-1095. DOI: 10.1002/jmv.24737

[10] Hau PM, Lung HL, Wu M, Tsang CM, Wong KL, Mak NK et al. Targeting Epstein-Barr virus in nasopharyngeal carcinoma. Frontiers in Oncology. 2020;**10**:1-18. Available from: https://www.frontiersin.org/articles/10.3389/fonc.2020.00600. [Accessed: February 11, 2023]

[11] Ng WT, Chow JCH, Beitler JJ, Corry J, Mendenhall W, Lee AWM, et al. Current radiotherapy considerations for nasopharyngeal carcinoma. Cancers. 2022;**14**:5773. DOI: 10.3390/cancers14235773

[12] Miller BJ, Gupta G. Adenoidectomy. In: StatPearls. Treasure Island, FL: StatPearls Publishing; 2022. Available from: http://www.ncbi.nlm.nih.gov/books/NBK535352/. [Accessed: January 16, 2023]

[13] Arambula A, Brown JR, Neff L. Anatomy and physiology of the palatine tonsils, adenoids, and lingual tonsils. The World Journal of Otorhinolaryngology – Head & Neck Surgery. 2021;**7**:155-160. DOI: 10.1016/j.wjorl.2021.04.003

[14] Golla S. Chapter 5— Adenoidectomy. In: Myers EN,

Carrau RL, Eibling DE, Ferguson BJ, Ferris RL, Gillman GS, Golla S, Grandis JR, Hirsch BE, Johnson JT, Raz Y, Rosen CA, Schaitkin BM, Snyderman CH, Toh EH, editors. Oper. Otolaryngol. Head Neck Surg. Second ed. Philadelphia: W.B. Saunders; 2008. pp. 33-37. DOI: 10.1016/B978-1-4160-2445-3.50009-1

[15] Mnatsakanian A, Heil JR, Sharma S. Anatomy, head and neck, adenoids. In: StatPearls. Treasure Island, FL: StatPearls Publishing; 2022. Available from: http://www.ncbi.nlm.nih.gov/books/NBK538137/. [Accessed: January 18, 2023]

[16] Jaw TS, Sheu RS, Liu GC, Lin WC. Development of adenoids: A study by measurement with MR images. The Kaohsiung Journal of Medical Sciences. 1999;**15**:12-18

[17] Vogler RC, Ii FJ, Pilgram TK. Age-specific size of the normal adenoid pad on magnetic resonance imaging. Clinical Otolaryngology and Allied Sciences. 2000;**25**:392-395. DOI: 10.1046/j.1365-2273.2000.00381.x

[18] Zitelli BJ, McIntire SC, Nowalk AJ, Garrison J. Otolaryngology. In: Zitelli and Davis' Atlas of Pediatric Physical Diagnosis. E-Book. 8th ed. Philadelphia: Elsevier Inc.; 2021. Available from: https://www.clinicalkey.com/#!/content/book/3-s2.0-B9780323393034000244 [Accessed: January 18, 2023]

[19] Nicodemo J, Hamersley E, Baker P, Reed S. Benign adenoidal hypertrophy caused by adenovirus presenting as a nasopharyngeal mass concerning for malignancy. International Journal of Pediatric Otorhinolaryngology. 2020;**138**:110300. DOI: 10.1016/j.ijporl.2020.110300

[20] Li H, Wang H, Hao H, An H, Geng H. Influences of airway obstruction caused by adenoid hypertrophy on growth and development of craniomaxillofacial structure and respiratory function in children. Computational and Mathematical Methods in Medicine. 2022;**2022**:5096406. DOI: 10.1155/2022/5096406

[21] Marieb EN, Hoehn K. Human Anatomy & Physiology. 9th ed. Boston: Pearson; 2013

[22] Chan KH, Abzug MJ, Liu AH. 26—Sinusitis. In: Leung DYM, Szefler SJ, Bonilla FA, Akdis CA, Sampson HA, editors. Pediatr. Allergy Princ. Pract. Third ed. London: Elsevier; 2016. pp. 228-237.e3. DOI: 10.1016/B978-0-323-29875-9.00026-4

[23] Moideen SP, Mytheenkunju R, Govindan Nair A, Mogarnad M, Afroze MKH. Role of adenoid-nasopharyngeal ratio in assessing adenoid hypertrophy. Indian Journal of Otolaryngology and Head & Neck Surgery. 2019;**71**:469-473. DOI: 10.1007/s12070-018-1359-7

[24] Zhao T, Zhou J, Yan J, Cao L, Cao Y, Hua F, et al. Automated adenoid hypertrophy assessment with lateral cephalometry in children based on artificial intelligence. Diagnostics. 2021;**11**:1386. DOI: 10.3390/diagnostics11081386

[25] Onal M, Onal O, Turan A. Can secondary lymphoid organs exert a favorable effect on the mild course of COVID-19 in children? Acta Oto-Laryngologica, Stockholm. 2020:1-2. DOI: 10.1080/00016489.2020.1814965

[26] Chang ET, Ye W, Zeng Y-X, Adami H-O. The evolving epidemiology of nasopharyngeal carcinoma. Cancer Epidemiology, Biomarkers & Prevention. 2021;**30**:1035-1047. DOI: 10.1158/1055-9965.EPI-20-1702

[27] McDermott AL, Dutt SN, Watkinson JC. The aetiology of nasopharyngeal carcinoma. Clinical Otolaryngology and Allied Sciences. 2001;**26**:82-92. DOI: 10.1046/j.1365-2273.2001.00449.x

[28] Sinha S, Gajra A. Nasopharyngeal cancer. In: StatPearls. Treasure Island, FL: StatPearls Publishing; 2022. Available from: http://www.ncbi.nlm.nih.gov/books/NBK459256/. [Accessed: January 19, 2023]

[29] Tang L, Chen Y, Chen C, Chen M, Chen N, Chen X, et al. The Chinese Society of Clinical Oncology (CSCO) clinical guidelines for the diagnosis and treatment of nasopharyngeal carcinoma. Cancer Communications. 2021;**41**:1195-1227. DOI: 10.1002/cac2.12218

[30] Guo R, Mao Y-P, Tang L-L, Chen L, Sun Y, Ma J. The evolution of nasopharyngeal carcinoma staging. The British Journal of Radiology. 2019;**92**:20190244. DOI: 10.1259/bjr.20190244

[31] Zhang Q, Wang Y, Yang S, Wu Q, Qiang W. What is the appropriate skin cleaning method for nasopharyngeal cancer radiotherapy patients? A randomized controlled trial. Supportive Care in Cancer. 2022;**30**:3875-3883. DOI: 10.1007/s00520-022-06835-8

[32] Lee HM, Okuda KS, González FE, Patel V. Current perspectives on nasopharyngeal carcinoma. Adv. Exp. Med. Biol. 2019;**1164**:11-34. DOI: 10.1007/978-3-030-22254-3_2

[33] Iseh K, Abdullahi A, Malami S. Clinical and histological characteristics of nasopharyngeal cancer in Sokoto, North Western, Nigeria. West African Journal of Medicine. 2009;**28**:151-155. DOI: 10.4314/wajm.v28i3.48438

[34] Xie S-H, Yu IT-S, Tse L-A, Mang OW, Yue L. Sex difference in the incidence of nasopharyngeal carcinoma in Hong Kong 1983-2008: Suggestion of a potential protective role of oestrogen. European Journal of Cancer. 2013;**1990**(49):150-155. DOI: 10.1016/j.ejca.2012.07.004

[35] Flores AD, Dickson RI, Riding K, Coy P. Cancer of the nasopharynx in British Columbia. American Journal of Clinical Oncology. 1986;**9**:281-291. DOI: 10.1097/00000421-198608000-00002

[36] Hamilton SN, Ho C, Laskin J, Zhai Y, Mak P, Wu J. Asian versus non-Asian outcomes in nasopharyngeal carcinoma: A north American population-based analysis. American Journal of Clinical Oncology. 2016;**39**:575-580. DOI: 10.1097/COC.0000000000000091

[37] Petersson F. Nasopharyngeal carcinoma: A review. Seminars in Diagnostic Pathology. 2015;**32**:54-73. DOI: 10.1053/j.semdp.2015.02.021

[38] Chua MLK, Wee JTS, Hui EP, Chan ATC. Nasopharyngeal carcinoma. The Lancet. 2016;**387**:1012-1024. DOI: 10.1016/S0140-6736(15)00055-0

[39] Buzatto GP, Tamashiro E, Proenca-Modena JL, Saturno TH, Prates MC, Gagliardi TB, et al. The pathogens profile in children with otitis media with effusion and adenoid hypertrophy. PLoS One. 2017;**12**:e0171049. DOI: 10.1371/journal.pone.0171049

[40] Chang K-H, Jun B-C, Jeon E-J, Park Y-S. Functional evaluation of paratubal muscles using electromyography in patients with chronic unilateral tubal dysfunction. European Archives of Oto-Rhino-Laryngology. 2013;**270**:1217-1221. DOI: 10.1007/s00405-012-2091-7

[41] Bhat V, Mani IP, Aroor R, Saldanha M, Goutham MK, Pratap D. Association of asymptomatic otitis media with effusion in patients with adenoid hypertrophy. Journal of Otology. 2019;**14**:106-110. DOI: 10.1016/j.joto.2018.12.001

[42] Sogebi OA, Oyewole EA, Ogunbanwo O. Asymptomatic otitis media with effusion in children with adenoid enlargement. Journal of the National Medical Association. 2021;**113**:158-164. DOI: 10.1016/j.jnma.2020.08.005

[43] Havas T, Lowinger D. Obstructive adenoid tissue: An indication for powered-shaver adenoidectomy. Archives of Otorhinolaryngology-Head & Neck Surgery. 2002;**128**:789-791. DOI: 10.1001/archotol.128.7.789

[44] Berkiten G, Kumral TL, Yildirim G, Uyar Y, Atar Y, Salturk Z. Eight years of clinical findings and biopsy results of nasopharyngeal pathologies in 1647 adult patients: A retrospective study. B-ENT. 2014;**10**:279-284

[45] Mankowski NL, Bordoni B. Anatomy, head and neck, nasopharynx. In: StatPearls. Treasure Island, FL: StatPearls Publishing; 2022. Available from: http://www.ncbi.nlm.nih.gov/books/NBK557635/. [Accessed: February 14, 2023]

[46] Stambuk HE, Patel SG, Mosier KM, Wolden SL, Holodny AI. Nasopharyngeal carcinoma: Recognizing the radiographic features in children. American Journal of Neuroradiology. 2005;**26**:1575-1579

[47] Lomaeva I, Aghajanyan A, Dzhaparidze L, Gigani OB, Tskhovrebova LV, Gigani OO, et al. Adenoid hypertrophy risk in children carriers of G-1082A polymorphism of IL-10 infected with human herpes virus (HHV6, EBV, CMV). Life. 2022;**12**:266. DOI: 10.3390/life12020266

[48] Shuaibu I, Usman M, Ajiya A, Chitumu D, Mohammed I, Abdullahi H, et al. Adenoid and tonsil hypertrophy in Zaria, North Western Nigeria: Review of clinical presentation and surgical outcome. Journal of the West African College of Surgeons. 2022;**12**:23. DOI: 10.4103/jwas.jwas_71_22

[49] Surov A, Ryl I, Bartel-Friedrich S, Wienke A, Kösling S. MRI of nasopharyngeal adenoid hypertrophy. The Neuroradiology Journal. 2016;**29**:408-412. DOI: 10.1177/1971400916665386

[50] Cassano M, De Corso E, Fiore V, Giancaspro R, Moffa A, Casale M, et al. Update of endoscopic classification system of adenoid hypertrophy based on clinical experience on 7621 children. Acta Otorhinolaryngologica Italica. 2022;**42**:257-264. DOI: 10.14639/0392-100X-N1832

[51] Maheswaran S, Rupa V, Ebenezer J, Manoharan A, Irodi A. Relative etiological importance of adenoid hypertrophy versus sinusitis in children with persistent rhinorrhoea. Indian Journal of Otolaryngology and Head & Neck Surgery. 2015;**67**:34-38. DOI: 10.1007/s12070-014-0743-1

[52] Shokouhi F, Jahromi AM, Majidi MR, Salehi M. Montelukast in adenoid hypertrophy: Its effect on size and symptoms. Iranian Journal of Otorhinolaryngology. 2015;**27**:443

[53] Dixit Y, Tripathi PS. Community level evaluation of adenoid hypertrophy on the basis of symptom scoring and its X-ray correlation. Journal of Family Medicine and Primary Care. 2016;**5**:789

[54] Zwierz A, Domagalski K, Masna K, Burduk P. Effectiveness of evaluation

of adenoid hypertrophy in children by flexible nasopharyngoscopy examination (FNE), proposed schema of frequency of examination: Cohort study. Diagnostics. 2022;**12**:1734. DOI: 10.3390/diagnostics12071734

[55] Mlynarek A, Tewfik MA, Hagr A, Manoukian JJ, Schloss MD, Tewfik TL, et al. Lateral neck radiography versus direct video rhinoscopy in assessing adenoid size. The Journal of Otolaryngology. 2004;**33**:360-365. DOI: 10.2310/7070.2004.03074

[56] Kindermann CA, Roithmann R, Lubianca Neto JF. Sensitivity and specificity of nasal flexible fiberoptic endoscopy in the diagnosis of adenoid hypertrophy in children. International Journal of Pediatric Otorhinolaryngology. 2008;**72**:63-67. DOI: 10.1016/j.ijporl.2007.09.013

[57] Zhang X, Li H, Liu X, Zhang Q, Liu H, Wang X, et al. [Study and analysis on the quantitative detection of EBV-DNA in adenoidal hypertrophic and tonsillitis tissues of children], Lin Chuang Er Bi Yan Hou Tou Jing Wai Ke Za Zhi. Journal of Clinical Otorhinolaryngology. 2009;**23**:1108-1111

[58] Bofares KM. Epstein-Barr virus infection as significant predisposing factor and post-radiotherapy prognostic indicator among Libyan patients with nasopharyngeal cancer. Journal of Biomedical Research & Environmental Sciences. 2022;**3**:1020-1026. DOI: 10.37871/jbres1548

[59] Feng Q, Liang J, Wang L, Ge X, Ding Z, Wu H. A diagnosis model in nasopharyngeal carcinoma based on PET/MRI radiomics and semiquantitative parameters. BMC Medical Imaging. 2022;**22**:150. DOI: 10.1186/s12880-022-00883-6

[60] Raica V, Bratu A, Zaharia C, Salcianu I. CT evaluation of squamous cell carcinoma of the nasopharynx. Current Health Sciences Journal. 2019;**45**:79-86. DOI: 10.12865/CHSJ.45.01.11

[61] Liu Z, Li H, Yu KJ, Xie S-H, King AD, Ai Q-YH, et al. Comparison of new magnetic resonance imaging grading system with conventional endoscopy for the early detection of nasopharyngeal carcinoma. Cancer. 2021;**127**:3403-3412. DOI: 10.1002/cncr.33552

[62] Shayah A, Wickstone L, Kershaw E, Agada F. The role of cross-sectional imaging in suspected nasopharyngeal carcinoma. Annals of the Royal College of Surgeons of England. 2019;**101**:325-327. DOI: 10.1308/rcsann.2019.0025

[63] Ji MF, Sheng W, Cheng WM, Ng MH, Wu BH, Yu X, et al. Incidence and mortality of nasopharyngeal carcinoma: Interim analysis of a cluster randomized controlled screening trial (PRO-NPC-001) in southern China. Annals of Oncology. 2019;**30**:1630-1637. DOI: 10.1093/annonc/mdz231

[64] Wang KH, Austin SA, Chen SH, Sonne DC, Gurushanthaiah D. Nasopharyngeal carcinoma diagnostic challenge in a nonendemic setting: Our experience with 101 patients. The Permanente Journal. 2017;**21**:16-180. DOI: 10.7812/TPP/16-180

[65] King AD, Woo JKS, Ai QY, Chan JSM, Lam WKJ, Tse IOL, et al. Complementary roles of MRI and endoscopic examination in the early detection of nasopharyngeal carcinoma. Annals of Oncology. 2019;**30**:977-982. DOI: 10.1093/annonc/mdz106

[66] King AD, Vlantis AC, Bhatia KSS, Zee BCY, Woo JKS, Tse GMK, et al. Primary nasopharyngeal carcinoma:

Diagnostic accuracy of MR imaging versus that of endoscopy and endoscopic biopsy. Radiology. 2011;**258**:531-537. DOI: 10.1148/radiol.10101241

[67] King AD, Vlantis AC, Tsang RKY, Gary TMK, Au AKY, Chan CY, et al. Magnetic resonance imaging for the detection of nasopharyngeal carcinoma. American Journal of Neuroradiology. 2006;**27**:1288-1291

[68] Gao Y, Zhu S-Y, Dai Y, Lu B-F, Lu L. Diagnostic accuracy of sonography versus magnetic resonance imaging for primary nasopharyngeal carcinoma. Journal of Ultrasound in Medicine. 2014;**33**:827-834. DOI: 10.7863/ultra.33.5.827

[69] Chen Y, Xin X, Cui Z, Zheng Y, Guo J, Chen Y, et al. Diagnostic value of serum Epstein-Barr virus capsid antigen-IgA for nasopharyngeal carcinoma: A meta-analysis based on 21 studies. Clinical Laboratory. 2016;**62**:1155-1166. DOI: 10.7754/clin.lab.2015.151122

[70] Cheng Y, Bai L, Shang J, Tang Y, Ling X, Guo B, et al. Preliminary clinical results for PET/MR compared with PET/CT in patients with nasopharyngeal carcinoma. Oncology Reports. 2020;**43**:177-187. DOI: 10.3892/or.2019.7392

[71] Chan S-C, Yeh C-H, Yen T-C, Ng S-H, Chang JT-C, Lin C-Y, et al. Clinical utility of simultaneous whole-body 18F-FDG PET/MRI as a single-step imaging modality in the staging of primary nasopharyngeal carcinoma. European Journal of Nuclear Medicine and Molecular Imaging. 2018;**45**:1297-1308. DOI: 10.1007/s00259-018-3986-3

[72] Cai Y-L, Li J, Lu A-Y, Zheng Y-M, Zhong W-M, Wang W, et al. Diagnostic significance of combined detection of Epstein-Barr virus antibodies, VCA/IgA, EA/IgA, Rta/IgG and EBNA1/IgA for nasopharyngeal carcinoma. Asian Pacific Journal of Cancer Prevention. 2014;**15**:2001-2006. DOI: 10.7314/APJCP.2014.15.5.2001

[73] Cengiz K, Kumral TL, Yıldırım G. Diagnosis of pediatric nasopharynx carcinoma after recurrent adenoidectomy. Case Reports in Otolaryngology. 2013;**2013**:653963. DOI: 10.1155/2013/653963

[74] Geiger Z, Gupta N. Adenoid hypertrophy. In: StatPearls. Treasure Island, FL: StatPearls Publishing; 2022. Available from: http://www.ncbi.nlm.nih.gov/books/NBK536984/. [Accessed: January 20, 2023]

[75] Sorin C, Min S, Carino G. Patient with prior COVID-19 infection presenting with acute upper airway obstruction: A case report. Cureus. 2022;**14**:1-5. DOI: 10.7759/cureus.23214

[76] France AJ, Kean DM, Douglas RH, Chiswick OM, St Clair D, Best JJ, et al. Adenoidal hypertrophy in HIV-infected patients. The Lancet (London, Englera). 1988;**2**:1076. DOI: 10.1016/s0140-6736(88)90092-x

[77] Olsen WL, Jeffrey RB, Sooy CD, Lynch MA, Dillon WP. Lesions of the head and neck in patients with AIDS: CT and MR findings. American Journal of Roentgenology. 1988;**151**:785-790. DOI: 10.2214/ajr.151.4.785

[78] Rout MR, Mohanty D, Vijaylaxmi Y, Bobba K, Metta C. Adenoid hypertrophy in adults: A case series. Indian Journal of Otolaryngology and Head & Neck Surgery. 2013;**65**:269-274. DOI: 10.1007/s12070-012-0549-y

[79] Rajeshwary A, Rai S, Somayaji G, Pai V. Bacteriology of symptomatic adenoids in children, north. The

American Journal of the Medical Sciences. 2013;**5**:113-118. DOI: 10.4103/1947-2714.107529

[80] Boll DT, Haaga JR. CT and MRI of the Whole Body. Philadelphia, PA: Elsevier; 2017

[81] Gao W, Li J, Li Q, An S. CYSLTR1 promotes adenoid hypertrophy by activating ERK1/2. Experimental and Therapeutic Medicine. 2018;**16**:966-970. DOI: 10.3892/etm.2018.6282

[82] Zhang J, Sun X, Zhong L, Shen B. IL-32 exacerbates adenoid hypertrophy via activating NLRP3-mediated cell pyroptosis, which promotes inflammation. Molecular Medicine Reports. 2021;**23**:226. DOI: 10.3892/mmr.2021.11865

[83] Atilla MH, Özdaş S, Özdaş T, Baştimur S, Muz SE, Öz I, et al. Association of Ugrp2 gene polymorphisms with adenoid hypertrophy in the pediatric population. Brazilian Journal of Otorhinolaryngology. 2018;**84**:599-607

[84] Babademez MA, Özdaş T, Özdaş S. The common genetic variants of toll-like receptor and susceptibility to adenoid hypertrophy: A hospital-based cohort study. The Turkish Journal of Medical Sciences. 2016;**46**:1449-1458

[85] Saedi B, Sadeghi M, Mojtahed M, Mahboubi H. Diagnostic efficacy of different methods in the assessment of adenoid hypertrophy. American Journal of Otolaryngology. 2011;**32**:147-151

[86] Shabaldina EV, Shabaldin AV, Riazantsev SV, Simbirtsev SV. The role of cytokine gene polymorphisms in the development of hypertrophy of the tonsils of the lymphoid pharyngeal ring and atopic march in the children. Vestnik Otorinolaringologica. 2013;**6**:18-23

[87] Centre international de recherche sur le cancer, editor. A review of human carcinogens. Lyon: International Agency for Research on Cancer; 2012

[88] Chan JK. Virus-associated neoplasms of the nasopharynx and sinonasal tract: Diagnostic problems. Modern Pathology. 2017;**30**:S68-S83. DOI: 10.1038/modpathol.2016.189

[89] Lo KW, To KF, Huang DP. Focus on nasopharyngeal carcinoma. Cancer Cell. 2004;**5**:423-428

[90] Pathmanathan R, Prasad U, Sadler R, Flynn K, Raab-Traub N. Clonal proliferations of cells infected with Epstein–Barr virus in preinvasive lesions related to nasopharyngeal carcinoma. The New England Journal of Medicine. 1995;**333**:693-698

[91] Svajdler M, Kaspirkova J, Mezencev R, Laco J, Torday T, Dubinsky P, et al. Human papillomavirus and Epstein-Barr virus in nasopharyngeal carcinoma in a non-endemic eastern European population. Neoplasma. 2016;**63**:107-114. DOI: 10.4149/neo_2016_013

[92] Yeung WM, Zong YS, Chiu CT, Chan KH, Sham JS, Choy DT, et al. Epstein-Barr virus carriage by nasopharyngeal carcinoma in situ. International Journal of Cancer. 1993;**53**:746-750

[93] Bossi P, Chan AT, Licitra L, Trama A, Orlandi E, Hui EP, et al. Nasopharyngeal carcinoma: ESMO-EURACAN clinical practice guidelines for diagnosis, treatment and follow-up. Annals of Oncology. 2021;**32**:452-465. DOI: 10.1016/j.annonc.2020.12.007

[94] Stenmark MH, McHugh JB, Schipper M, Walline HM, Komarck C, Feng FY, et al. Nonendemic HPV-positive nasopharyngeal carcinoma: Association

with poor prognosis. International Journal of Radiation Oncology, Biology, Physics. 2014;**88**:580-588. DOI: 10.1016/j.ijrobp.2013.11.246

[95] Chang ET, Liu Z, Hildesheim A, Liu Q, Cai Y, Zhang Z, et al. Active and passive smoking and risk of nasopharyngeal carcinoma: A population-based case-control study in southern China. American Journal of Epidemiology. 2017;**185**:1272-1280. DOI: 10.1093/aje/kwx018

[96] Turati F, Bravi F, Polesel J, Bosetti C, Negri E, Garavello W, et al. Adherence to the Mediterranean diet and nasopharyngeal cancer risk in Italy. Cancer Causes & Control. 2017;**28**:89-95. DOI: 10.1007/s10552-017-0850-x

[97] Sernia S, Di Folco F, Altrudo P, Sbriccoli B, Sestili C, Colamesta V, et al. Risk of nasopharyngeal cancer, leukemia and other tumors in a cohort of employees and students potentially exposed to (FA) formaldehyde in university laboratories. La Clinica Terapeutica. 2016;**167**:43-47

[98] Siew SS, Kauppinen T, Kyyrönen P, Heikkilä P, Pukkala E. Occupational exposure to wood dust and formaldehyde and risk of nasal, nasopharyngeal, and lung cancer among Finnish men. Cancer Management and Research. 2012;**4**:223-232. DOI: 10.2147/CMAR.S30684

[99] Siew SS, Martinsen JI, Kjaerheim K, Sparén P, Tryggvadottir L, Weiderpass E, et al. Occupational exposure to wood dust and risk of nasal and nasopharyngeal cancer: A case-control study among men in four nordic countries—With an emphasis on nasal adenocarcinoma. International Journal of Cancer. 2017;**141**:2430-2436

[100] Xie S-H, Yu IT, Tse LA, Au JSK, Lau JSM. Occupational risk factors for nasopharyngeal carcinoma in Hong Kong Chinese: A case-referent study. International Archives of Occupational and Environmental Health. 2017;**90**:443-449

[101] Bei J-X, Li Y, Jia W-H, Feng B-J, Zhou G, Chen L-Z, et al. A genome-wide association study of nasopharyngeal carcinoma identifies three new susceptibility loci. Nature Genetics. 2010;**42**:599-603

[102] Chin Y-M, Mushiroda T, Takahashi A, Kubo M, Krishnan G, Yap L-F, et al. HLA-A SNPs and amino acid variants are associated with nasopharyngeal carcinoma in Malaysian Chinese. International Journal of Cancer. 2015;**136**:678-687

[103] Cui Q, Feng Q-S, Mo H-Y, Sun J, Xia Y-F, Zhang H, et al. An extended genome-wide association study identifies novel susceptibility loci for nasopharyngeal carcinoma. Human Molecular Genetics. 2016;**25**:3626-3634

[104] Ng CC, Yew PY, Puah SM, Krishnan G, Yap LF, Teo SH, et al. A genome-wide association study identifies ITGA9 conferring risk of nasopharyngeal carcinoma. Journal of Human Genetics. 2009;**54**:392-397

[105] Tsao SW, Yip YL, Tsang CM, Pang PS, Lau VMY, Zhang G, et al. Etiological factors of nasopharyngeal carcinoma. Oral Oncology. 2014;**50**:330-338. DOI: 10.1016/j.oraloncology.2014.02.006

[106] Tse K-P, Su W-H, Chang K-P, Tsang N-M, Yu C-J, Tang P, et al. Genome-wide association study reveals multiple nasopharyngeal carcinoma-associated loci within the HLA region at chromosome 6p21. 3. American Journal of Human Genetics. 2009;**85**:194-203

[107] Hildesheim A, Wang C-P. Genetic predisposition factors and nasopharyngeal carcinoma risk: A review of epidemiological association studies, 2000-2011: Rosetta stone for NPC: Genetics, viral infection, and other environmental factors. Seminars in Cancer Biology. 2012;**22**:107-116. DOI: 10.1016/j.semcancer.2012.01.007

[108] Choudhari SM, Shrivastav S. Comparative evaluation of adenoids and airway space in 12 to 14-year-old children with different growth patterns using cephalometric methods commonly used by ENT specialists. The Journal of Indian Orthodontic Society. 2022;**56**:23-28. DOI: 10.1177/0301574220966875

[109] Baldassari CM, Choi S. Assessing adenoid hypertrophy in children: X-ray or nasal endoscopy? The Laryngoscope. 2014;**124**:1509-1510. DOI: 10.1002/lary.24366

[110] Cassano P, Gelardi M, Cassano M, Fiorella ML, Fiorella R. Adenoid tissue rhinopharyngeal obstruction grading based on fiber endoscopic findings: A novel approach to therapeutic management. International Journal of Pediatric Otorhinolaryngology. 2003;**67**:1303-1309. DOI: 10.1016/j.ijporl.2003.07.018

[111] Chien C-Y, Chen A-M, Hwang C-F, Su C-Y. The clinical significance of adenoid-choanae area ratio in children with adenoid hypertrophy. International Journal of Pediatric Otorhinolaryngology. 2005;**69**:235-239. DOI: 10.1016/j.ijporl.2004.09.007

[112] Kubba H, Bingham BJ. Endoscopy in the assessment of children with nasal obstruction. The Journal of Laryngology and Otology. 2001;**115**:380-384. DOI: 10.1258/0022215011907929

[113] Parikh SR, Coronel M, Lee JJ, Brown SM. Validation of a new grading system for endoscopic examination of adenoid hypertrophy. Otolaryngology—Head and Neck Surgery. 2006;**135**:684-687. DOI: 10.1016/j.otohns.2006.05.003

[114] Wang DY, Clement PA, Kaufman L, Derde MP. Chronic nasal obstruction in children. A fiberscopic study. Rhinology. 1995;**33**:4-6

[115] Ysunza A, Pamplona MC, Ortega JM, Prado H. Video fluoroscopy for evaluating adenoid hypertrophy in children. International Journal of Pediatric Otorhinolaryngology. 2008;**72**:1159-1165. DOI: 10.1016/j.ijporl.2008.03.022

[116] Zicari AM, Rugiano A, Ragusa G, Savastano V, Bertin S, Vittori T, et al. The evaluation of adenoid hypertrophy and obstruction grading based on rhinomanometry after nasal decongestant test in children. European Review for Medical and Pharmacological Sciences. 2013;**17**:2962-2967

[117] Narang VP, Loroch A, Sambiagio G. Versatility and benefits of 4.0mm flexible nasal endoscopy in 118 children up to 10 years of age. Cureus. 2022;**14**:e22656. DOI: 10.7759/cureus.22656

[118] Handelman CS, Osborne G. Growth of the nasopharynx and adenoid development from one to eighteeen years. The Angle Orthodontist. 1976;**46**:243-259

[119] Holmberg H, Linder-Aronson S. Cephalometric radiographs as a means of evaluating the capacity of the nasal and nasopharyngeal airway. American Journal of Orthodontics. 1979;**76**:479-490

[120] Maw AR, Jeans WD, Fernando DCJ. Inter-observer variability in the clinical and radiological assessment of adenoid size, and the correlation with adenoid

volume. Clinical Otolaryngology and Allied Sciences. 1981;**6**:317-322

[121] McNamara JA. A method of cephalometric evaluation. American Journal of Orthodontics. 1984;**86**(6):449-469

[122] Caylakli F, Hizal E, Yilmaz I, Yilmazer C. Correlation between adenoid-nasopharynx ratio and endoscopic examination of adenoid hypertrophy: A blind, prospective clinical study. International Journal of Pediatric Otorhinolaryngology. 2009;**73**:1532-1535. DOI: 10.1016/j.ijporl.2009.07.018

[123] Elwany S. The adenoidal-nasopharyngeal ratio (A-N ratio)—Its validity in selecting children for adenoidectomy. The Journal of Laryngology and Otology. 1987;**101**:569-573

[124] Kurien M, Lepcha A, Mathew J, Ali A, Jeyaseelan L. X-rays in the evaluation of adenoid hypertrophy: It's role in the endoscopic ERA. Indian Journal of Otolaryngology and Head and Neck Surgery. 2005;**57**:45-47. DOI: 10.1007/BF02907627

[125] Lertsburapa K, Schroeder JW, Sullivan C. Assessment of adenoid size: A comparison of lateral radiographic measurements, radiologist assessment, and nasal endoscopy. International Journal of Pediatric Otorhinolaryngology. 2010;**74**:1281-1285. DOI: 10.1016/j.ijporl.2010.08.005

[126] Fujioka M, Young LW, Girdany BR. Radiographic evaluation of adenoidal size in children: Adenoidal-nasopharyngeal ratio. American Journal of Roentgenology. 1979;**133**:401-404

[127] Major MP, Saltaji H, El-Hakim H, Witmans M, Major P, Flores-Mir C. The accuracy of diagnostic tests for adenoid hypertrophy. Journal of the American Dental Association (1939). 2014;**145**:247-254. DOI: 10.14219/jada.2013.31

[128] Patel A, Brook CD, Levi JR. Comparison of adenoid assessment by flexible endoscopy and mirror exam. International Journal of Pediatric Otorhinolaryngology. 2020;**134**:110073. DOI: 10.1016/j.ijporl.2020.110073

[129] Asante D-B, Asmah RH, Adjei AA, Kyei F, Simpong DL, Brown CA, et al. Detection of human papillomavirus genotypes and Epstein-Barr virus in nasopharyngeal carcinomas at the Korle-Bu teaching hospital, Ghana. Scientific World Journal. 2017;**2017**:e2721367. DOI: 10.1155/2017/2721367

[130] Chan KCA, Woo JKS, King A, Zee BCY, Lam WKJ, Chan SL, et al. Analysis of plasma Epstein–Barr virus DNA to screen for nasopharyngeal cancer. The New England Journal of Medicine. 2017;**377**:513-522. DOI: 10.1056/NEJMoa1701717

[131] Li H-P, Hsu C-L, Chang Y-S. Screening of nasopharyngeal carcinoma using plasma Epstein-Barr virus DNA for at-risk population. Annals of Nasopharynx Cancer. 2018;**2**:1-3. DOI: 10.21037/anpc.2018.03.01

[132] Liu W, Chen G, Gong X, Wang Y, Zheng Y, Liao X, et al. The diagnostic value of EBV-DNA and EBV-related antibodies detection for nasopharyngeal carcinoma: A meta-analysis. Cancer Cell International. 2021;**21**:164. DOI: 10.1186/s12935-021-01862-7

[133] Chen H, Chi P, Wang W, Li L, Luo Y, Fu J, et al. Evaluation of a semi-quantitative ELISA for IgA antibody against Epstein-Barr virus capsid antigen in the serological diagnosis of nasopharyngeal carcinoma. International Journal of Infectious

Diseases. 2014;**25**:110-115. DOI: 10.1016/j.ijid.2014.03.1373

[134] Chen H, Zhong Q, Wu X, Ding Y, Chen Q, Xue N, et al. Preliminary evaluation of a candidate international reference for Epstein–Barr virus capsid antigen immunoglobulin a in China. Infectious Agents and Cancer. 2020;**15**:25. DOI: 10.1186/s13027-020-00294-8

[135] Li S, Deng Y, Li X, Chen Q, Liao X, Qin X. Diagnostic value of Epstein-Barr virus capsid antigen-IgA in nasopharyngeal carcinoma: A meta-analysis. Chinese Medical Journal. 2010;**123**:1201-1205

[136] Sham JS, Wei WI, Zong YS, Choy D, Guo YQ, Luo Y, et al. Detection of subclinical nasopharyngeal carcinoma by fibreoptic endoscopy and multiple biopsy. Lancet (London, England). 1990;**335**:371-374. DOI: 10.1016/0140-6736(90)90206-k

[137] Gorolay VV, Niles NN, Huo YR, Ahmadi N, Hanneman K, Thompson E, et al. MRI detection of suspected nasopharyngeal carcinoma: A systematic review and meta-analysis. Neuroradiology. 2022;**64**:1471-1481. DOI: 10.1007/s00234-022-02941-w

[138] King AD. MR imaging of nasopharyngeal carcinoma. Magnetic Resonance Imaging Clinics of North America. 2022;**30**:19-33. DOI: 10.1016/j.mric.2021.06.015

[139] Loh LE, Chee TS, John AB. The anatomy of the fossa of Rosenmuller—Its possible influence on the detection of occult nasopharyngeal carcinoma. Singapore Medical Journal. 1991;**32**:154-155

[140] Gao Y, Liu J-J, Zhu S-Y, Yi X. The diagnostic accuracy of ultrasonography versus endoscopy for primary nasopharyngeal carcinoma. PLoS One. 2014;**9**:e90412. DOI: 10.1371/journal.pone.0090412

[141] Aktas E, Sahin B, Ciledag N, Arda KN, Caglar E, Ilhan IE. Magnetic resonance imaging findings in childhood period nasopharynx cancer. Polish Journal of Radiology. 2015;**80**:555-560. DOI: 10.12659/PJR.895315

[142] Wu Y-P, Cai P-Q, Tian L, Xu J-H, Mitteer RA, Fan Y, et al. Hypertrophic adenoids in patients with nasopharyngeal carcinoma: Appearance at magnetic resonance imaging before and after treatment. Chinese Journal of Cancer. 2015;**34**:130-136. DOI: 10.1186/s40880-015-0005-y

[143] Liu Z, Chen Y, Su Y, Hu X, Peng X. Nasopharyngeal carcinoma: Clinical achievements and considerations among treatment options. Frontiers in Oncology. 2021;**11**:1-11. Available from: https://www.frontiersin.org/articles/10.3389/fonc.2021.635737; [Accessed: February 11, 2023]

[144] Jiromaru R, Nakagawa T, Yasumatsu R. Advanced nasopharyngeal carcinoma: Current and emerging treatment options. Cancer Management and Research. 2022;**14**:2681-2689. DOI: 10.2147/CMAR.S341472

[145] Cabezas-Camarero S, Pérez-Segura P. Liquid biopsy in head and neck cancer: Current evidence and future perspective on squamous cell, salivary gland, paranasal sinus and nasopharyngeal cancers. Cancers. 2022;**14**:2858. DOI: 10.3390/cancers14122858

[146] Asante D-B, Calapre L, Ziman M, Meniawy TM, Gray ES. Liquid biopsy in ovarian cancer using circulating tumor DNA and cells: Ready for prime time? Cancer Letters. 2020;**468**:59-71. DOI: 10.1016/j.canlet.2019.10.014

Chapter 6

Benign and Malignant Tumors of the Tonsils

Anusha Vaddi, Shravan Renapurkar and Sonam Khurana

Abstract

Tonsils are lymphoid tissues in the oral cavity and nasopharyngeal region arranged in Waldeyer's ring. The Waldeyer's ring consists of pairs of pharyngeal (adenoids), tubal, palatine, and lingual tonsils. These are usually hyperplastic at a younger age and decrease with age. However, asymmetric enlargement might be a sign of pathology. It could be due to tonsillitis, abscess, and benign tumors, such as fibromas, teratomas, and angiomas such as lymphangioma, hemangioma, and inclusion cyst. Benign tumors of the tonsils are usually rare but not uncommon. It could be due to malignancies such as lymphoma, squamous cell carcinoma, or metastasis. This chapter focuses on clinical, histopathological and radiographic features of benign and malignant tumors of palatine and lingual tonsils.

Keywords: lingual tonsil, palatine tonsil, tonsillar carcinoma, tonsillar tumor, classification of tonsillar tumors

1. Introduction

Tonsils are developed from the second branchial cleft. This location corresponds to the intersection of oral epiblast and intestinal hypoblast. According to embryology,

Benign tumors	Malignant tumors
Fibroma	Squamous cell carcinoma
Lymphangioma/lymphoid polyp	Lymphoma—Hodgkin's and Non-Hodgkin's
Squamous cell papilloma	Mucoepidermoid carcinoma
Lipoma	Adenocarcinoma, adenoid cystic carcinoma
Fibroxanthoma (histiocytoma)	Melanoma
Chondromas	Sarcomas: Embryonal rhabdomyosarcoma Synovial sarcoma Angiosarcoma Kaposi's sarcoma
Mixed tumor (pleomorphic adenoma)	Metastatic malignancies
Oncocytoma, ganglioneuroma, neurilemmoma pigmented nevus, hamartoma	Plasmacytoma (extramedullary)

Table 1.
Benign and malignant tumors of lingual and palatine tonsil [1].

IntechOpen

an organ formed from combining two different tissues has more potential for neoplastic growth [2]. Although benign and malignant tumors of the tonsillar region are more common, there is very scarce literature regarding the definitive classification of tonsillar tumors. In the WHO classification of tumors of the oropharynx, tonsillar tumors are included along with the base of the tongue and adenoids. This chapter focuses exclusively on palatine and lingual tonsillar tumors. These tumors are comprehensively classified according to the histologic nature of the lesion (**Table 1**).

2. Benign tumors of tonsils

Benign tumors of the tonsils are rarer than malignant tumors. Most benign tumors of the tonsils are reported in the younger age group. Most patients are asymptomatic, and a benign tumor is often detected as an incidental finding. Other clinical symptoms include the presence/sense of mass, sore throat, and difficulty swallowing/breathing. Most benign tumors of the tonsil manifest in the form of a polyp, and clinical signs and symptoms are identical. The histopathological examination provides a definitive diagnosis of the lesion based on the tissue of origin. **Table 1** provides a list of benign tumors. The clinical features of common benign tonsillar tumors are discussed below.

2.1 Hamartomatous fibrous polyps/fibro-epithelial polyp/tonsillar fibroma

These present as a polypoid mass attached to the tonsil. It may be sessile/pedunculated (**Figure 1**). The patient recognizes mass after it attains a specific size and interferes with functional movements such as deglutition. The most common

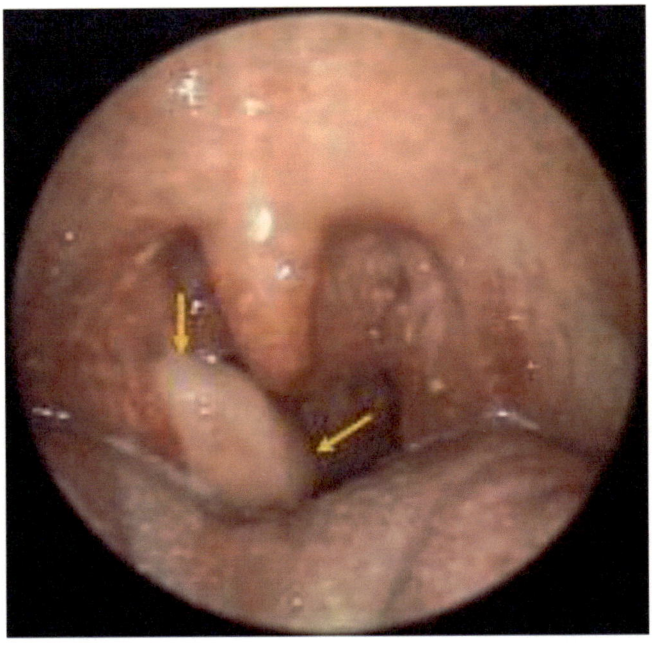

Figure 1.
Well-defined, smooth-surfaced fibroepithelial polyp (yellow arrows) arising from the superior pole of the right palatine tonsil [3]. Source: https://www.ncbi.nlm.nih.gov/pmc/articles/PMC8556748/. License: https://creativecommons.org/licenses/by/4.0/.

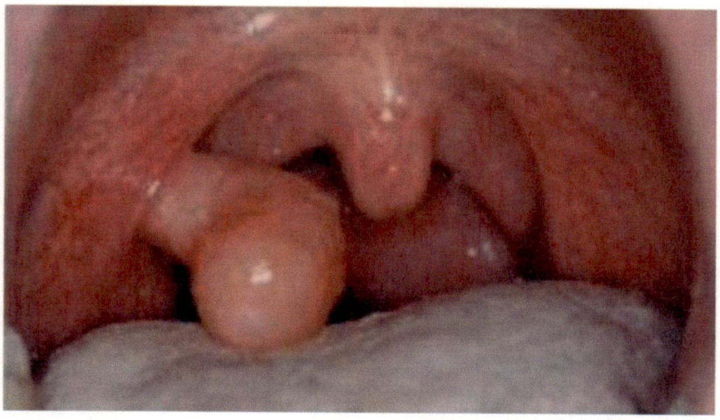

Figure 2.
Pedunculated polyp of lymphoid origin in the right palatine tonsil [4]. Source: https://www.hindawi.com/journals/crim/2011/183182/. License: http://creativecommons.org/licenses/by/3.0/.

clinical features include pale pink color, lymphadenopathy, and asymptomatic lesion. However, patients might present with cough or foreign body sensation. Reports of airway obstruction due to benign tonsillar mass are scarce. The rate of malignant transformation is significantly less.

Histopathology: Most tonsillar fibromas demonstrate stratified squamous epithelium with fibrous/collagenous stroma.

2.2 Lymphoid tonsillar mass/Lymphangiomatous polyp

Lymphangiomatous polyps are congenital tumors of the lymphatic system. They are hamartomatous malformations. They are present at birth or manifest in early life (**Figure 2**). The clinical presentation would be similar to a fibroma. Bilateral occurrence is rare, although few cases are reported in the literature [5].

Histopathology: Foci of well-organized lymphoid tissue would be present within the tonsillar mass.

2.3 Papilloma

It is one of the common benign neoplasms of the tonsil. Clinically they present as grayish-white exophytic lesions with a wrinkled surface. The lesions may be either sessile/pedunculated.

Histopathology: Papilloma has characteristic, multiple finger-like projections with hyperplastic squamous epithelium and fibrovascular core.

2.4 Lipoma

Lipomas are mesenchymal tumors of fat cells. They are seen less frequently in the head and neck region, especially the tonsillar area. They are benign, slow-growing tumors. The clinical presentation would be similar to other benign tumors. Lipomas can be lobulated. Extensive lipoma might cause airway obstruction.

Imaging: Lipomas have characteristic computed tomography (CT) and Magnetic Resonance imaging (MRI) features. In CT imaging, they appear as well-defined, non-enhancing low, attenuation homogeneous lesions (**Figure 3**). MRI demonstrates a hyperintense lesion on both T1-weighted (T1W) and T2-weighted (T2W) images.

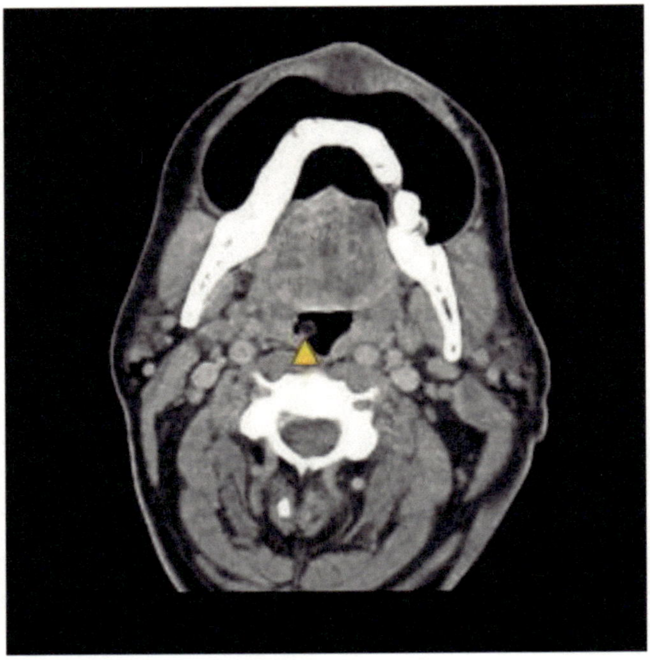

Figure 3.
Axial section of contrast-enhanced CT demonstrating a pedunculated lipoma arising from right palatine tonsil. Notice the non-enhancement of the lesion [6]. Source: https://www.eurorad.org/case/17083. License: http://creativecommons.org/licenses/by-nc-sa/4.0/.

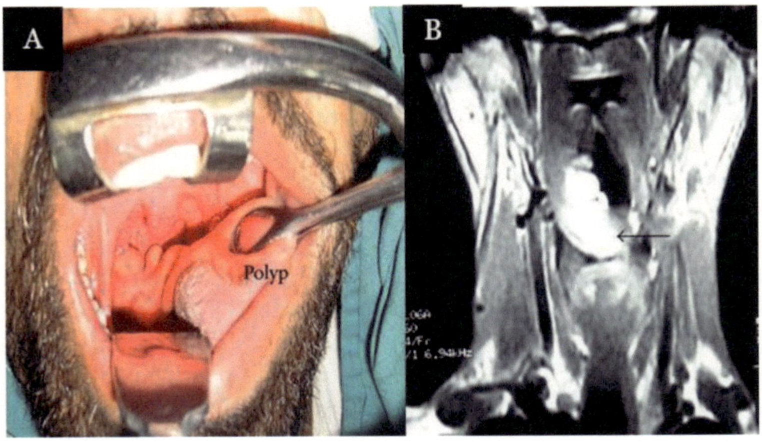

Figure 4.
Clinical presentation of tonsillar lipoma (A) and coronal section of T2-weighted MRI image demonstrating hyperintense lesion (B) [7]. Source: https://www.hindawi.com/journals/crim/2014/480130/. License: http://creativecommons.org/licenses/by/3.0/.

Loss of the signal is evident in Fat-saturated images and STIR sequences. Both CT and MRI post-contrast images do not demonstrate enhancement of the lesion (**Figure 4**).

Histopathology: Adipose tissue divided into lobules with collagenous septa and interspersed vascular channels. Histologically there are different variants of lipoma, such as fibro lipoma, chondrolipoma, and myolipoma.

2.5 Management of Benign tumors of tonsils

Most benign tumors, such as lipoma, fibroma, papilloma, and lymphangioma, present as polypoid masses. Tonsillectomy and surgical excision of the lesion, followed by histopathologic examination, is the most common treatment option. The definitive diagnosis is based on the predominant tissue in the excised specimen. Few cases can be managed with the excision of polypoid mass without tonsillectomy, especially if the polypoid mass is pedunculated [7]. There is less chance for recurrence and malignant transformation of benign tumors of the tonsils. The prognosis is usually good for benign tumors.

3. Malignant tumors of tonsils

Oropharyngeal (OP) cancers include tumors arising from the palatine tonsil, the base of the tongue, the walls of the pharynx, and the soft palate. Palatine tonsils constitute lymphoid tissue embedded in the tonsillar fossa located in the lateral walls of the oropharynx between the tonsillar pillars. Palatine tonsils cancers comprise tumors of the anterior and posterior tonsillar pillar, tonsillar fossa, and plica triangularis. The lingual tonsil constitutes lymphoid tissue in the base of the tongue. Lingual tonsillar cancers comprise tumors of the base of the tongue.

Tonsilar squamous cell carcinomas (SCC) are the most common malignant tonsillar neoplasms, followed by non-Hodgkin's lymphoma. Most oropharyngeal SCCs (OPSCC) are associated with human papillomavirus (HPV). Tobacco, smoking habits, iron deficiency, avitaminosis, and syphilis have been implicated as other etiology factors for tonsillar neoplasms. The overall incidence of Head and neck SCC (HNSCC) has been reducing since the 1980s due to declining smoking. However, there is a rapid increase in human papillomavirus (HPV) induced OPSCC in younger patients [8].

The presenting symptoms for most tonsillar neoplasms are sore throat, local pain, and the sensation of a mass in the neck. The tonsillar growth begins as a superficial granular ulcer in the tonsillar region. Eventually, the ulcer erodes the surface. They produce a submucosal mass with or without surface ulceration. Tonsillar tumors might spread to alveolar ridges and buccal mucosa. Tonsillar neoplasms metastasize to uni/bilateral lymph nodes and present as lymphadenopathy. Radiating pain in the ear is characteristic of advanced tonsillar malignancy. During initial medical diagnosis, most malignant tonsillar tumors are in advanced stages or extended beyond the tonsil. The poor tactile sensation in the tonsillar region compared to the oral cavity could be the reason for the occult nature of tonsillar malignancies [9].

Both carcinomas and lymphomas present as asymmetric enlargements of the tonsil. It is challenging to differentiate from clinical examination. Some lymphomas present as bilateral tonsillar masses. There is conflicting literature regarding the excision of unilateral asymmetric enlarged tonsils without other suspicious features of malignancy. However, a tumor should always be considered in the differential diagnosis of these cases, and judicious follow-up is recommended [10].

3.1 Squamous cell carcinoma (SCC)

Due to the inherent lack of afferent lymphatic channels, carcinoma in the tonsils is likely a primary malignancy rather than metastasis [11].

Tonsillar pillar SCC: The most common locations for primary tonsillar SCC are the anterior tonsillar pillar and the tonsils. The palatoglossus muscle forms the anterior tonsillar pillar. The anterior tonsillar pillar tumors may spread to masticator space. In such cases, patients might experience pain and trismus due to the involvement of pterygoid muscles. The tumor can spread anterolaterally to involve pharyngeal constrictors, pterygomandibular raphe, and retromolar trigone region of the oral cavity. The anterior tonsillar pillars drain into the level I, II, and III nodes. The majority of patients will have nodal involvement at the initial presentation.

The palatopharyngeus muscle forms the posterior tonsillar pillar. Tumors in this region can spread to the soft palate, thyroid cartilage, pterygomandibular raphe, and oral cavity. The posterior tonsillar pillar drains only into level II nodes. But if a tumor spreads to the oropharynx, this region drains into level V and retropharyngeal nodes [12].

Tonsillar fossa SCC: Tumors of the tonsillar fossa are often occult. In this region, the tumor can spread to the parapharyngeal, carotid, and masticator space, the tonsillar pillars, and the gnathic region. The tonsillar fossa drains into the level I to IV nodes.

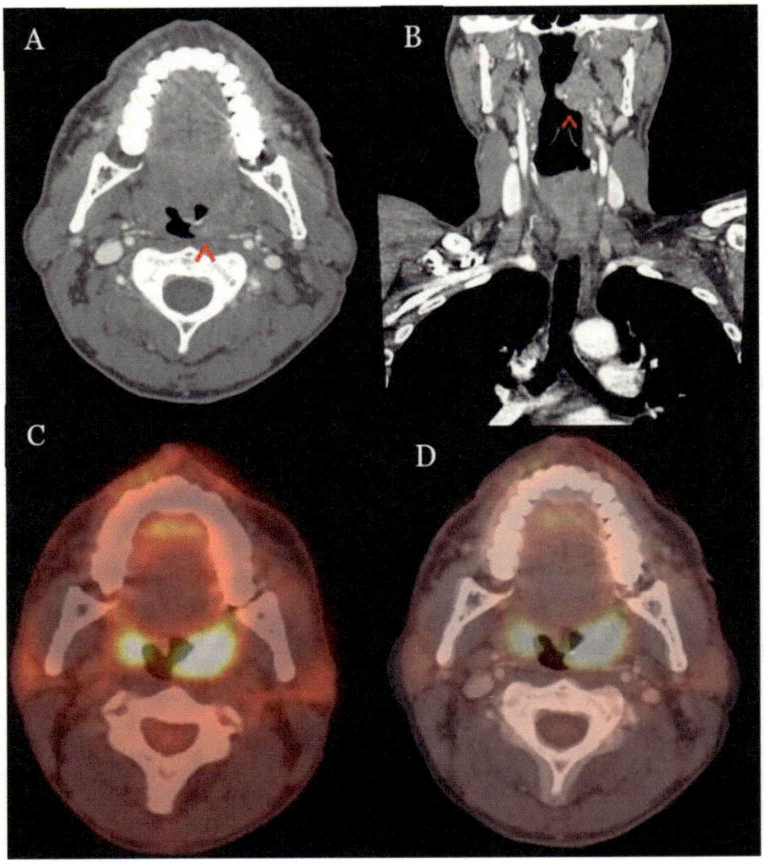

Figure 5.
*Bilateral tonsillar squamous cell carcinoma [13]: (A) Axial CT neck with contrast demonstrating left palatine tonsillar mass (red arrowhead) extending towards the midline; (B) Sagittal CT neck with contrast showing the medial extension of mass (red arrowhead) towards the uvula within the oropharynx; (C) Fluorodeoxyglucose (FDG) PET/CT axial view demonstrating increased radiotracer uptake in both the left and right palatine tonsils. But no soft tissue abnormality right palatine tonsil was noted in CT (**Figure 5A** and **B**); and (D) PET/Ct superimposed at 55% opacity for improved visualization of tumor margins in the oropharynx. Source: https://onlinelibrary.wiley.com/doi/10.1002/cnr2.1615. License: http://creativecommons.org/licenses/by/4.0/.*

CT Imaging: A small squamous cell carcinoma lesion is difficult to delineate from the surrounding normal tissues on CT imaging. The large lesions are usually exophytic and invasive. The contrast-enhanced CT (CECT) typically presents with heterogeneous uptake. Positron emission tomography (PET)/CT imaging demonstrates the extent of the tumor and helps in treatment planning (**Figure 5**). If there is nodal involvement, the node appears enlarged, often round with central necrosis or entirely cystic.

MRI Imaging: The typical characteristic of SCC is enlarged tonsils that appear isointense to hypointense on T1W images relative to normal lymphoid tissues. These characteristics on T1W make it challenging to differentiate from muscles. On T2W images, the tumor appears hyperintense, which helps to distinguish it from surrounding lymphoid tissues. On T1W with gadolinium administration, the tumors show marked enhancement due to the uptake of the contrast. Most often, tumors are diagnosed when they progress to stage 3 or 4. The reason for delayed diagnosis could be normal asymmetric variation in the shape and contour of the tonsils. It is generally hard to differentiate tonsillitis from an early malignancy, including carcinoma and lymphoma. The advanced stage SCC can invade adjacent anatomical structures such as the pharyngeal wall, palate, and tongue base, which helps differentiate from benign lesions. Contrast-enhanced MRI can differentiate malignant lesions due to their superior soft tissue resolution [14].

Histopathology: The epithelium of tonsils originates from ectoderm, and mesoderm and lymphocytes are populated in the crypts. The epithelial lining of both palatine and lingual tonsils and crypts is the stratified squamous epithelium and ciliated pseudostratified columnar for the pharyngeal tonsils. The origin of HPV and non-HPV-associated SCC is different. The SCC associated with HPV originates from the epithelium lining the crypts, whereas non-HPV originates from the tonsillar surface epithelium. The characteristic feature of SCC is squamous differentiation and invasion of the basement membrane. Due to invasion, it can extend to underlying tissues along with desmoplastic stromal reaction and inflammatory infiltrate. The inflammatory cells mainly include lymphocytes and plasma cells. The most common SCC are moderately-differentiated variants, showing nuclear pleomorphism and mitosis and less keratinization than the well-differentiated variety. The poorly differentiated type has predominantly immature cells with typical and atypical mitoses, less keratinization, and rarely necrosis [15].

Management: The treatment is based on the size of the tumor. Recently, Trans Oral Robotic Surgery (TORS) is a popular treatment option, followed by neck dissection and radiotherapy for nodal involvement. The T1 or T2 tumors are usually treated with chemotherapy, radiotherapy, and TORS with nodal dissection. Large tumors with extensive nodal involvement are mainly treated with chemoradiotherapy [15].

3.2 Lymphoma

Lymphoma accounts for the second most common malignancies of the head and neck. Most head and neck lymphomas are Hodgkin, and only 5% are non-Hodgkin. The tonsils are the most common site of non-Hodgkin lymphoma (NHL) in the head and neck region. The clinical symptoms of primary non-Hodgkin lymphoma of the tonsils include a sore throat or feeling of a lump in the throat, lymphadenopathy, dysphagia, and occasionally systemic symptoms such as fever, weight loss, and night sweats. It usually has a rapid onset with a short clinical course of a few weeks and predominantly occurs in the older age group.

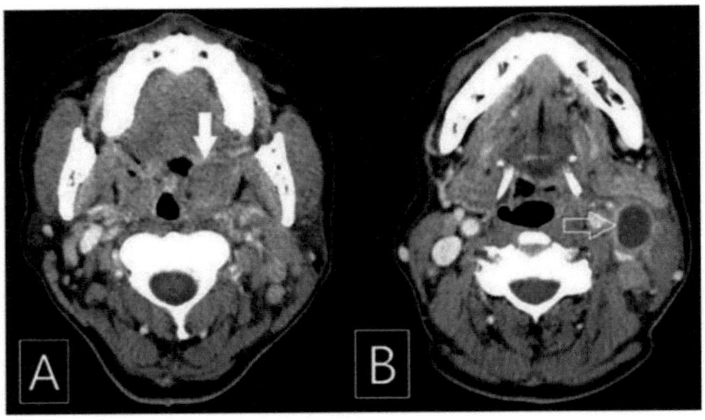

Figure 6.
Contrast-enhanced CT (CECT) scan of the patient. (A) Hypertrophic and slightly enhanced left palatine tonsil (solid arrow) and (B) enlarged ipsilateral cervical lymph node demonstrating central low attenuated lesion (arrow) [16]. Source: https://synapse.koreamed.org/articles/1129387. License: http://creativecommons.org/licenses/by-nc/4.0/34:78-82.

CT Imaging: On CT soft tissue window with contrast, lymphoma has a slightly homogenous enhancement, with density higher than muscle (**Figure 6**). In contrast to NHL, SCC shows heterogeneous enhancement due to necrosis and invasion of adjacent structures [17].

MRI Imaging: The T1W images show homogenous intermediate signals similar to normal tonsillar tissues, mild hyperintensity on T2, and minimal gadolinium enhancement on T1 contrast. The occasional, mild heterogeneous signal indicates areas of focal necrosis. Because signals of NHL are similar to normal tonsillar tissues, MRI is not a reliable imaging modality. MRI is primarily used to locate the tumor and detect nodal metastasis. Tonsillar lymphoma has a higher incidence of cervical node metastasis. Like SCC, lymphomas present as a round or lobulated exophytic mass. But unlike SCC, most lymphoma displaces adjacent structures rather than invasion. On an MRI, the presence of a large tumor that displaces the adjacent structure instead of invasion is highly suggestive of lymphoma [18].

Histopathology: According to WHO classification [19], 66–75% of lymphomas noted in the Waldeyer's ring are diffuse large B-cell types. The other types, such as small lymphocytic, follicular large cell, lymphoblastic, Burkitt's lymphoma, and peripheral T Cell types are rare.

Management: The treatment protocol is dependent upon the stage of the disease. The treatment includes radiotherapy alone or combined therapy for stages I and II occurring in the Waldeyer's ring. The radiotherapy targets anatomic sites, including the nasopharynx, bilateral tonsils, soft palate, hard palate, and the root of the tongue. The lymph nodes included are cervical, supra, and sub-clavicular. Combined radio and chemotherapy improve the 5 years prognosis. For stages III and IV, chemotherapy is the primary treatment. The prognosis depends on the stage and whether the tumor is primary or recurrent. The low-grade NHL has a better prognosis, whereas recurrent and/or intermediate/high-stage NHL might recur beyond the primary site. Currently, combined chemo and radiotherapy are universally accepted treatment modalities [16].

3.3 Mucoepidermoid carcinoma (MEC)

It is the most common primary salivary gland malignancy. It can occur in the minor salivary glands of the palatine tonsils. Patients might present with

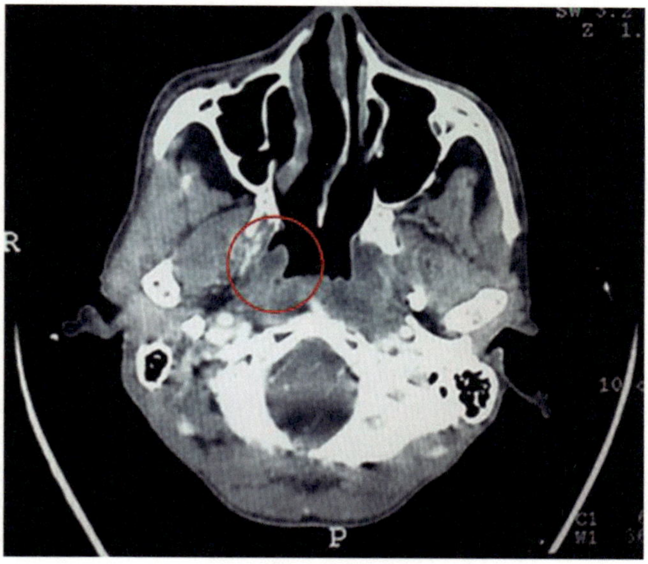

Figure 7.
Axial CT image demonstrating solid lesion of MEC with lobulated and ill-defined margins [20]. Source: https://www.hindawi.com/journals/crionm/2015/827560/. License: http://creativecommons.org/licenses/by/3.0/.

asymptomatic swelling that eventually progresses to an ulcerated mass. Few tumors present as fluctuant masses with a blue or red hue identical to mucocele.

CT Imaging: On CECT, low-grade lesions appear heterogeneous with well-defined margins. The mucous deposits show low-intensity areas similar to cysts. High-grade lesions have infiltrative, ill-defined margins with heterogeneous contrast uptake and nodal metastasis (**Figure** 7).

MRI Imaging: On T1W, low-grade lesions appear heterogeneous, well-defined mass with mainly low signals, and high-grade mass shows intermediate signals with infiltrative margins. On T1W with contrast, the lesion shows heterogeneous uptake with no uptake by mucous deposits. On T2W, the mucous deposits show hyperintense signals, like cysts. Low-grade lesions have heterogeneous signals, and high-grade lesions have intermediate signals with infiltrative margins.

Histopathology: Histopathology of palatine MEC demonstrates fragments of oral mucosa with non-keratinized stratified squamous epithelium showing dysplastic features such as atypia and mitotic figures. The lamina propria reveals features of glandular origin. A combination of mucous-producing cells and epidermoid (squamous cells). An intermediate progenitor cell is found in some cases. Immunohistochemistry is also a valuable diagnostic tool for salivary gland tumors.

Management: Tonsillectomy with total tumor excision is the treatment of choice for MEC. Some cases might require radical tonsillectomy and ipsilateral neck dissection based on the extent of the lesion. In advanced-stage cases, chemo and radiotherapy are used before or after surgery [20].

3.4 Adenocarcinomas

Most of the adenocarcinomas in the palatine tonsils are metastatic from the lung and gastrointestinal tract. In recent times, the number of tonsillar carcinomas associated with HPV 16 has increased, and most of them were SCC. There are few case reports of HPV p16-positive adenocarcinomas. HPV-associated adenocarcinomas occur in younger patients. They comprise less than 1% of all malignancies of palatine tonsils.

Imaging: Like other malignancies of the tonsillar region, CT and MRI are helpful in locating the extent and treatment plan of the adenocarcinoma. In one case report, standardized uptake values (SUVs) of the radiotracer were 14.2 for the tonsillar mass and 7.2 for retropharyngeal nodes in the initial PET scan. There was adenopathy of the cervical lymph nodes.

Histopathology: A few case reports have demonstrated tumor mass made up of glandular and cribriform structures centered around the tonsillar crypts. The cancer cells have a basaloid appearance with pleomorphic nuclei. Along with pleomorphic nuclei, vesicular chromatin and inconspicuous nucleoli were also noted. Sometimes cells grow in cystic spaces. Infiltration into underlying bone or muscle is noted in some cases. Perineural invasion can occur. Immunohistochemical staining helps in distinguishing adenocarcinomas from other salivary gland tumors.

Management: HPV-associated adenocarcinoma responds more to radiotherapy or surgery and has a better prognosis than non-HPV lesions. Usually, tonsillar cancers are diagnosed at advanced stages after distant metastasis. In such cases, extensive neck dissection with adjuvant chemo-radiotherapy has better outcomes. Immunotherapy has a good influence on the prognosis of tonsillar carcinomas [21, 22].

3.5 Melanoma

Primary mucosal melanoma accounts for 1.3% of cases in the head and neck region. In descending order, the primary sites in the head and neck region include the nose and paranasal sinuses, oral cavity, pharynx, and larynx. The oropharynx is not a common site of mucosal melanoma. Mucosal melanoma is more common in males than females; the average age is 61–65. Melanoma usually has a poor prognosis, so an early diagnosis has a better outcome.

Imaging: For diagnosis of melanoma, MRI is the modality of choice. The imaging features of MRI are more sophisticated than CT densities (**Figure 8**). The characteristic features of melanoma on MRI are attributed to melanotic pigment and hemorrhage within the lesion. T1W has hyperintense signals and hypointense on T2W due to the paramagnetic properties of melanin and free radicals produced by the metals within the

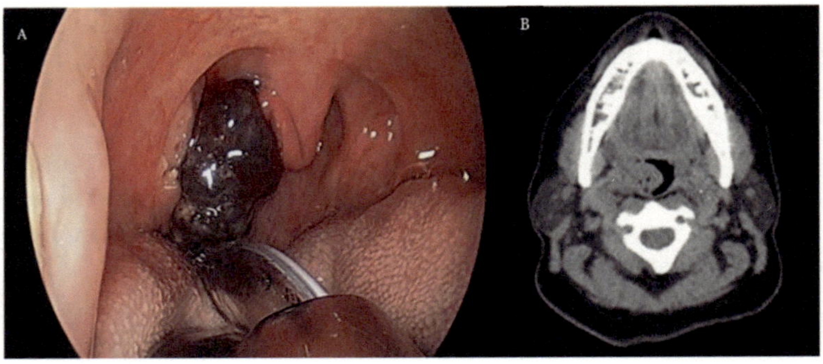

Figure 8.
(A) Clinical image demonstrating extensive, pigmented exophytic lesion (metastasis to palatine tonsil from a cutaneous melanoma); and (B) Non-contrast CT axial section demonstrating exophytic right tonsillar mass [23]. Source: https://academic.oup.com/jscr/article/2022/2/rjac022/6524980. License: https://creativecommons.org/licenses/.

pigment. Metastasis due to primary mucosal melanoma is difficult to diagnose. PET/CT helps assess the suspected metastasis due to the high fluorodeoxyglucose avidity.

Histopathology: Primary mucosal melanoma has the characteristic presence of proliferation of malignant melanocytes. The malignant melanocytes have variable phenotypes, viz. plasmacytoid, spindle, and epithelioid cells with hyperchromatic nuclei with prominent nucleoli. The malignant cells display high mitosis and invasive patterns to submucosa and destroy underlying tissues. Mucosal melanoma with mixed cell phenotypes is more prone to metastasis and vascular invasion.

Management: The recent guidelines for the treatment of mucosal melanoma dictates that localized cases without distant metastasis should be removed surgically with negative margins. If margins are positive, adjuvant radiotherapy and immunotherapy are treatments of choice. For cases with distant metastasis, combination immunotherapy is the first line of treatment, and chemotherapy is the second line of treatment [24].

3.6 Sarcoma

Tonsillar sarcomas are not very common. Unlike tonsillar squamous cell carcinomas, sarcomas grow rapidly and spread through visceral metastasis. The etiopathogenesis of sarcoma is unknown. Detailed knowledge of tonsillar anatomy is important to understand sarcoma's signs and symptoms and decide on treatment. The superior boundary of the tonsils is formed by the junction of the soft palate and facial pillars and is inferiorly continuous as vallecula. Inferiorly, if lymphoid tissues are more, no line of distinction is present between facial and lingual tonsils. Tonsils are separated from the carotid sheath by the middle constrictor muscle of the pharynx. Tonsils are not directly attached to the anterior pillar or the plica triangularis. A fairly moderate size sarcoma at the superior aspect of the tonsils can cause displacement of the supratonsillar fossa. A larger mass at this site can cause displacement of the uvula and soft palate bulging. A large tumor mass at the inferior aspect can mimic an indurated fixed lymph node due to displacement of the tissues below the jaw angle. Tumor present between the superior and inferior extent (middle third) can be visualized by tongue depression.

Imaging: Computed tomography and magnetic resonance imaging (MRI) provides information about the extent and the tissue composition of sarcomas due to their heterogeneity in tissue types. For example, fibrosarcoma has intermediate intensities on both T1W and T2W images, and liposarcoma is hyperintense on T1 due to lipid component and intermediate on T2W. These modalities also help in the treatment planning and assessing the prognosis. Most tumors have clearly defined margins, either because of surrounding soft tissue planes or because of significantly different attenuation values from the surrounding soft tissue. On the CT scan, there was no correlation between the CT densities and the histologic type of the tumor (**Figure 9**).

Histopathology: Sarcomas are malignant mesenchymal tumors that are rare in the tonsillar region. Tonsils are composed of three different types of tissues, viz. Squamous epithelium, reticular connective tissues, and lymphocytes. Lymphocytes and supporting reticulum of lymphoid tissues tend to differentiate into sarcomas of tonsils. The most common tumor types include fibrous histiocytoma, leiomyosarcoma, liposarcoma, fibrosarcoma, synovial sarcoma, epithelioid sarcoma, hemangiopericytoma, lymphangiosarcoma, and follicular dendritic cell sarcoma. The histological features vary based on the grade, type, and site of the origin.

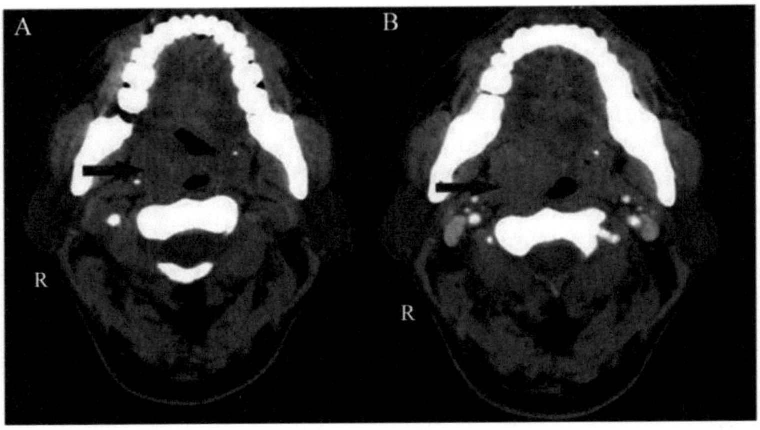

Figure 9.
(A) CT scan demonstrating a well-circumscribed, homogeneously enlarged 4.6 × 2.5 × 2.5-cm right tonsil; and (B) post-contrast image demonstrating slight continuing heterogeneous enhancement [25]. Source: https://www.spandidos-publications.com/10.3892/ol.2014.2726. License: https://creativecommons.org/licenses/by-nc-nd/4.0/.

Management: The mainstay of treatment of sarcomas is surgery, except in Ewing sarcoma and angiosarcoma cases. These sarcomas are responsive to chemoradiation or neoadjuvant chemotherapy. Larger size, metastasis, and positive margins have a poor prognosis. The sarcomas of the tonsils and/or head and neck region are a diverse group of malignant mesenchymal tumors. Their improved histological classification and combination treatment modalities are important to improve the prognosis and overall impact on the quality of life of the patients [26].

3.7 Metastatic malignancies

Metastasis to palatine tonsils is extremely rare. Only a few cases have been reported in the literature. The mechanism of metastasis is unclear. It could occur through the retrograde lymphatic spread, hematogenous or paravertebral plexus from lungs, or through direct inoculation of lung tumor through bronchoscopy. Physical examination might reveal swollen and edematous tonsils. The patient may have difficulty in breathing, pain, and discomfort. Tonsillar metastasis is often detected as an incidental finding during the routine oral examination. In some cases, the patient might have symptoms such as a sore throat and the sensation of a mass in the neck. Tonsillar metastasis can be uni/bi-lateral depending on the primary neoplasm [27].

Imaging: Imaging studies such as PET/CT are used to identify, diagnose, and stage metastasis to different organs.

Histopathology: Histopathology provides a definitive diagnosis and information on the primary tumor of origin (**Figure 10**).

Management: A combination of surgery, radiotherapy, and chemotherapy are the treatment options depending on the extent and primary tumor of origin. There is no definitive treatment for metastatic malignancy of the tonsils, and the prognosis is poor [28].

3.8 Extramedullary Plasmacytoma (EMP)

Plasmacytomas are malignancies of plasma cells that primarily involve bone. Sometimes, plasmacytomas occur in soft tissues, called extramedullary

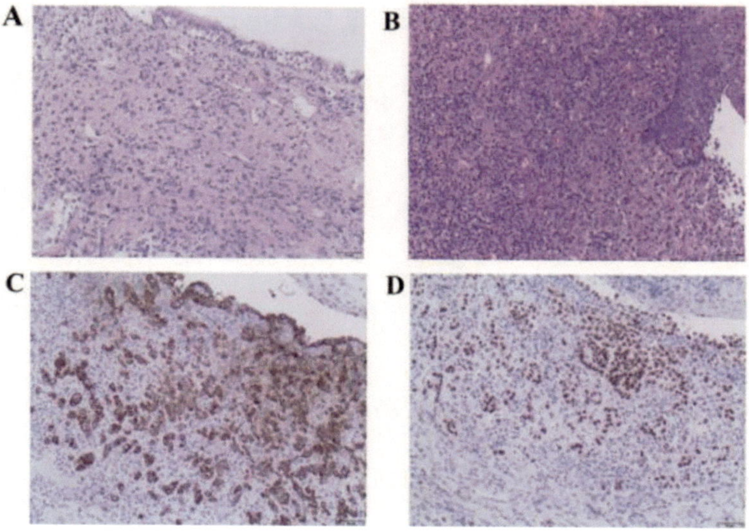

Figure 10.
(A) Respiratory columnar epithelium of the right medial main bronchus undermined by a poorly differentiated carcinoma with lymphovascular invasion hematoxylin and eosin staining (magnification, ×100); (B) Stratified squamous epithelium of the right palatine tonsil demonstrating histologically identical cancerous infiltrate (magnification, ×100); (C) Cytokeratin 7; and (D) thyroid transcription factor-1 positivity establish the diagnosis of metastatic pulmonary adenocarcinoma (magnification, ×100) [28]. Source: https://www.spandidos-publications.com/10.3892/mco.2018.1776. License: http://creativecommons.org/licenses/by/4.0/.

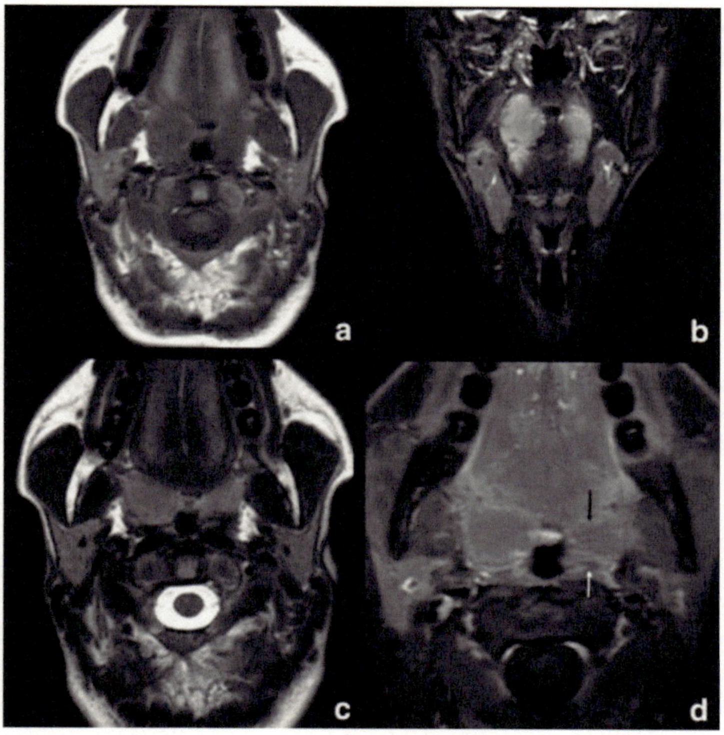

Figure 11.
Tonsillar plasmacytoma: (a) Axial non-contrast T1W; (b) coronal STIR; and (c) Axial T2W and d. postgadolinium T1W with fat saturation MR images. The arrow in image d demonstrates the obliteration of the right palatine tonsillar crypts combined with linear horizontal enhancement to the left [29].

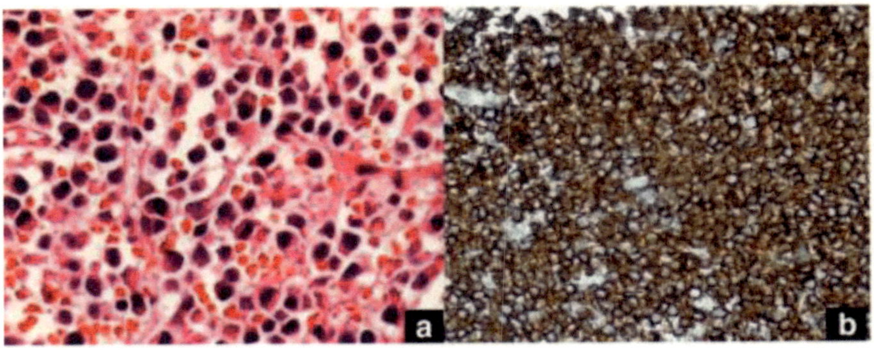

Figure 12.
(a) Plasma cells with an eccentric nucleus and abundant cytoplasm (hematoxylin–eosin × 40); and (b) Diffuse cytoplasmic, focal membranous CD138 staining on the plasma cells (streptavidin-biotin peroxidase × 400) [29]. Source: https://bmcmedimaging.biomedcentral.com/articles/10.1186/s12880-018-0261-9. License: http://creativecommons.org/licenses/by/4.0/.

plasmacytomas (EMP). These tumors are usually rare and occur mostly in the upper aerodigestive tract. EMPs are extremely rare in the tonsillar region. Clinical presentation includes painless mass, unilateral swelling in the tonsillar region, and lymphadenopathy. There are case reports of bilateral EMP. FNAC might be inconclusive in some cases due to difficulty in distinguishing from reactive lesions.

Imaging: CT, MRI, and PET/CT imaging provide information regarding the extent of the lesion (**Figure 11**).

Histopathology: Effacement of normal tonsillar architecture and diffuse infiltration of sheets of neoplastic cells with plasmacytoid morphology (eccentric nuclei, cart-wheel appearance of nuclear membrane) (**Figure 12**).

Management: Excisional biopsy of lesion for definitive diagnosis. Referral to a hematologist is recommended to rule out multiple myeloma. Solitary EMP is managed with a combination of surgery and radiotherapy. Periodic follow-up is recommended to monitor the recurrence and progression of the lesion as multiple myeloma [29].

4. Conclusion

Majority of benign tumors of the tonsils are managed with surgical excision of tumors with or without tonsillectomy. There is a low chance of recurrence and the prognosis is usually good for benign tumors. Early diagnosis and intervention determine the prognosis for malignant tonsillar tumors. The overall survival rate is better with HPV-positive tumors than with HPV-negative. The high survival rate in HPV-positive cases can be reduced by smoking. The other factors that help to improve prognosis include young age, localized tumor with lack of metastasis, and low comorbidities. CECT/MRI are recommended imaging modalities. The diagnosis of CECT sequences in the maxillofacial region is limited due to the streak artifact. The small primary mucosal tumors are difficult to diagnose; hence clinical evaluation is complimentary, and the thin CT sections help for better assessment. Underdiagnosing the primary lesion by failure to recognize invasion and lymph node metastasis can lead to poor prognosis. Careful evaluation of adjacent soft tissues and osseous structures, involvement of retropharyngeal lymph nodes on ipsilateral/contralateral sites, and detailed knowledge of anatomy are vital for better disease control and prognosis.

Conflict of interest

The authors declare no conflict of interest.

Author details

Anusha Vaddi[1]*, Shravan Renapurkar[2] and Sonam Khurana[3]

1 Oral Diagnostic Sciences, Virginia Commonwealth University School of Dentistry, Richmond, Virginia, USA

2 Oral and Maxillofacial Surgery, Virginia Commonwealth University School of Dentistry, Richmond, Virginia, USA

3 Department of Oral and Maxillofacial Pathology, Radiology and Medicine, New York University College of Dentistry, New York, USA

*Address all correspondence to: vaddia@vcu.edu

References

[1] Hyams VJ. Differential diagnosis of neoplasia of the palatine tonsil. Clinical Otolaryngology and Allied Sciences. 1978;**3**:117-126

[2] Hara HJ. Benign tumors of the tonsil: with special reference to fibroma. Archives of Otolaryngology. 1933;**1**:62-69

[3] Marini K, Garefis K, Skliris JP, Peltekis G, Astreinidou A, Florou V. Fibroepithelial polyp of palatine tonsil: A case report. The Pan African Medical Journal. 2021;**39**:276

[4] Balatsouras DG, Fassolis A, Koukoutsis G, Ganelis P, Kaberos A. Primary lymphangioma of the tonsil: A case report. Case Reports in Medicine. 2011;**2011**:31

[5] Gan W, Xiang Y, He X, Feng Y, Yang H, Liu H, et al. A CARE-compliant article: Lymphangiomatous polyps of the palatine tonsils in a miner: A case report. Medicine. 2019;**98**(1)

[6] Unzué G, Viteri G, Alberdi N, López P, de Llano L, Lage T, et al. Lipoma of palatine tonsil. Section head and neck imaging. Eurorad. 2020. DOI: 10.35100/eurorad/case.17083

[7] Kanotra SP, Davies J. Management of tonsillar lipoma: Is tonsillectomy essential? Case Reports in Otolaryngology. 2014;**2014**:4

[8] Filion E, Le QT. Oropharynx: Epidemiology and treatment outcome. In: Functional Preservation and Quality of Life in Head and Neck Radiotherapy. Berlin, Heidelberg: Springer; 2009. pp. 15-29

[9] Martin H, Sugarbaker EL. Cancer of the tonsil. The American Journal of Surgery. 1941;**52**(1):158-196

[10] Cinar F. Significance of asymptomatic tonsil asymmetry. Otolaryngology-Head and Neck Surgery. 2004;**131**(1):101-103

[11] Heffner DK. Pathology of the tonsils and adenoids. Otolaryngologic Clinics of North America. 1987;**20**(2):279-286

[12] Corey A. Pitfalls in the staging of cancer of the oropharyngeal squamous cell carcinoma. Neuroimaging Clinics. 2013;**23**(1):47-66

[13] Rossi NA, Reddy DN, Rawl JW, Dong J, Qiu S, Clement CG, et al. Synchronous tonsillar tumors with differing histopathology: A case report and review of the literature. Cancer Reports. 2022;**5**(9):e1615

[14] Weber AL, Romo L, Hashmi S. Malignant tumors of the oral cavity and oropharynx: Clinical, pathologic, and radiologic evaluation. Neuroimaging Clinics of North America. 2003;**13**(3):443-464. DOI: 10.1016/s1052-5149(03)00037-6

[15] Rousseau A, Badoual C. Head and Neck: Squamous cell carcinoma: An overview. Atlas of Genetics and Cytogenetics in Oncology and Haematology. Mar 2012;**16**(2):145-155

[16] Kim YC, Kwon M, Kim JP, Park JJ. A case of malignant lymphoma misdiagnosed as acute tonsillitis with subsequent lymphadenitis. Kosin Medical Journal. 2019;**34**(1):78-82

[17] Wang XY, Wu N, Zhu Z, Zhao YF. Computed tomography features of enlarged tonsils as the first symptom of non-Hodgkin's lymphoma. Chinese Journal of Cancer. 2010;**29**(5):556-560

[18] King AD, Lei KI, Ahuja AT. MRI of primary non-Hodgkin's lymphoma of

the palatine tonsil. The British Journal of Radiology. 2001;**74**(879):226-229

[19] Vardiman JW. The World Health Organization (WHO) classification of tumors of the hematopoietic and lymphoid tissues: An overview with emphasis on the myeloid neoplasms. Chemico-Biological Interactions. 19 Mar 2010;**184**(1-2):16-20

[20] Teixeira LN, Montalli VA, Teixeira LC, Passador-Santos F, Soares AB, Araújo VC. Mucoepidermoid carcinoma of the palatine tonsil. Case Reports in Oncological Medicine. 2015;**2015**:15

[21] Damato S, Thavaraj S, Winter S, Shah K. Human papillomavirus-associated adenocarcinoma of the palatine tonsil. Human Pathology. 2014;**45**(4):893-894

[22] Sethi A, Sundermann J, Neeta P. Human Papillomavirus induced adenocarcinoma of tonsil: A rare entity. Clinical Oncological Case Report. 2022;**5**:2

[23] Barton BM, Ramsey T, Magne JM, Worley NK. Delayed metastatic melanoma to the pharyngeal tonsil in an African American female. Ochsner Journal. 2019;**19**(2):181-183

[24] Manolidis S, Donald PJ. Malignant mucosal melanoma of the head and neck: A review of the literature and report of 14 patients. Cancer. 1997;**80**(8):1373-1386

[25] Lu ZJ, Li J, Zhou SH, Dai LB, Yan SX, Wu TT, et al. Follicular dendritic cell sarcoma of the right tonsil: A case report and literature review. Oncology Letters. 2015;**9**(2):575-582

[26] O'Neill JP, Bilsky MH, Kraus D. Head and neck sarcomas: Epidemiology, pathology, and management. Neurosurgery Clinics. 2013;**24**(1):67-78

[27] Bar R, Netzer A, Ostrovsky D, Daitzchman M, Golz A. Abrupt tonsillar hemorrhage from a metastatic hemangiosarcoma of the breast: Case report and literature review. Ear, Nose & Throat Journal. 2011;**90**(3):116-200

[28] Zaubitzer L, Rotter N, Aderhold C, Gaiser T, Jungbauer F, Kramer B, et al. Metastasis of pulmonary adenocarcinoma to the palatine tonsil. Molecular and Clinical Oncology. 2019;**10**(2):231-234

[29] Celebi İ, Bozkurt G, Polat N. Tonsillar Plasmacytoma: Clues on magnetic resonance imaging. BMC Medical Imaging. 2018;**18**(1):1-4